High Blood Pressure Lowered Naturally

By
Janice McCall Failes
and
Frank W. Cawood

 For information, or to order copies, mail $11.97 + $3.00 postage to:

FC&A Publishing
103 Clover Green
Peachtree City, Georgia 30269

First edition. Printed and bound by the Banta Company. Cover design by Debbie Williams.

Acknowledgments

To Andrew G. Aronfy, M.D., F.A.A.P. for your valuable contributions on the importance of monitoring blood pressure in children.

Thanks to two nurses who shared their experience with controlling high blood pressure. Judith Perkins, a public health nurse in Rockbridge County, Virginia gave me support and valuable statistics. Patsy Ford, a nurse in Hot Springs, Virginia, who helped with step-by-step directions on how to take your own blood pressure.

Prayers and thanks to our Stuanton District Volunteers in Mission team to Puerto Rico who shared Christ's love with me, prayed with me, and renew my spirit. Through you, I was drawn closer to our God who gave us these intricate bodies and the ability to love one another. Dios te bendiga.

To June Gunden, whose skills as an editor are unsurpassed.

To Alice Johnston, for your conscientiousness

and hard work in typesetting the manuscript.

To Debbie Williams, for your artwork and design.

To all the staff of FC&A for your support and help and, especially, thanks and praise to our Lord and Saviour, Jesus Christ, who gives us strength and the promise of eternal life.

Pleasant words are like a honey-comb, sweetness to the soul and health to the body.

-PROVERBS 16:24

For I will restore health to you, And your wounds will I heal, Says the Lord.

-JEREMIAH 20:17a

WARNING

High blood pressure is a serious disease. Check with your physician before discontinuing *any medication* or trying to treat yourself.

Table of Contents

Part One

Understanding High Blood Pressure

High blood pressure, or hypertension, is one of modern society's worst enemies. An estimated 60 million Americans have some form of this disease. It is a subtle condition, often with no obvious symptoms in its early stages, yet people with high blood pressure are three to five times more vulnerable to heart attacks than those with normal blood pressure.

Although it is rarely listed on death certificates as the cause of death, high blood pressure, if left untreated, can lead to numerous other causes of death. Strokes, heart attacks, kidney failure and blindness are major examples of the devastation of this elusive illness.

With all these complications, high blood pressure may be the nation's leading cause of death. However, 25 to 40 percent of all high blood pressure victims are unaware they have the disease. Education about its seriousness and its many known causes is half the battle against the disease.

The first part of this book, therefore, is an attempt to try to understand high blood pressure. What is it? Who is at greatest risk of getting it? How can you most accurately measure it? How serious is it?

It is only after we understand this dangerous enemy that we can begin to fight it effectively.

Chapter One

What Is High Blood Pressure?

Blood pressure is the force exerted on the walls of arteries, veins and capillaries as the heart pumps blood through the body. Without enough pressure, blood would not be able to pick up oxygen from the lungs or force impurities through the kidneys to the bladder. The body must always maintain enough blood pressure for essential functions.

Temporary hypertension is a normal rise in blood pressure to meet the body's needs in times of stress or increased bodily activity, such as digestion or exercise. Overeating, psychological stress and sudden hard exercise may cause brief, high jumps in blood pressure.

This form of hypertension becomes a problem if the body has been weakened by disease. Then, a temporary rise in blood pressure can cause a weak part of the body to fail. Self-training to recognize stressful situations and to relax is helpful. Some medical clinics have biofeedback programs which help people learn to relax and overcome temporary problems.

What is chronic high blood pressure?

Chronic high blood pressure occurs when continuous excessive pressure is placed on the walls of arteries as the heart pumps blood throughout the body. An individual with chronic high blood pressure may be calm, relaxed or even asleep, yet the force of blood running through the body is still too great.

In some rare cases, high blood pressure can be caused by another disease, like kidney artery disease, Cushings's disease, brain tumors, narrowing of the aorta (the main artery in the body), or tumors of the adrenal glands. Although these cases are rare, this is a reason why a doctor needs to examine anyone with blood pressure problems.This book does not attempt to explore these causes of high blood pressure, however, but concentrates on the more common causes.

What are the symptoms of high blood pressure?

The symptoms of high blood pressure are often silent. It may have no obvious symptoms in its early stages. Often, high blood pressure may be detected only by having the blood pressure taken. Later, as high blood pressure damages the body, many health problems may show up. Symptoms such as tiredness, insomnia, shortness of breath, flushing of the face, headaches, heart palpitations, dizziness, nervousness, nose bleed, temporary blindness or pain may be experienced. Since these traits are so general, and most people with normal blood pressure can experience them, the symptoms are not a reliable way to detect high blood pressure.

Forty percent of people with high blood pressure are unaware that they have it, according to statistics from the Virginia Department of Health. Twenty percent know but are not participating in therapy. Another twenty percent are receiving treatment, but their blood pressure isn't fully controlled. Only twenty percent of victims are aware that they have high blood pressure and have it under control through proper treatment.

You cannot *feel* that you have high blood pressure

— you must have your blood pressure checked regularly.

Chapter Two

Who Gets High Blood Pressure?

The exact cause of high blood pressure is a mystery in 80 to 90 percent of all cases. We know many of the factors that can lead to high blood pressure, but they may or may not affect a certain person.

For example, someone with a history of high blood pressure in his family who is overweight and smokes may not ever develop high blood pressure. Yet another person with few risk factors may have extremely high blood pressure. Usually though, most people can lower their blood pressure by changing the factors that can be controlled, even if they have other risk factors that they can't control.

This chapter will concentrate on the risk factors you can't control — such as heredity and age. The factors you can control — such as diet and lifestyle — will be the subject of Part Two of this book.

Heredity

Children who have one parent with high blood pressure have a greater chance of developing the disease than children with no family history of high blood pressure. When both parents have high blood pressure, the odds are even greater. Check out your parents' and their immediate family's health histories. If you are at high risk, you should take extra care in your diet, exercise program and lifestyle.

A new genetic screening test may eventually make it possible to identify people at risk for high blood pressure before clinical signs of disease appear, the *Medical World News* reports.

Researchers in California and Michigan have discovered "genetic markers" which signal "increased risk for hypertention and atherosclerosis," the article says.

Dr. Phillipe Frossard, project director at California Biotechnology, has identified 14 markers for hypertention so far, focusing on genes involved with regulating blood pressure. A link between the markers and hypertension is being studied in 70 high blood pressure patients and 30 with normal blood pressure at Cornell University Medical Center.

Frossard believes that genetic testing to predict high blood pressure in people with no symptoms will become routine within the next few years.

Not only will accurate prediction of high blood pressure and atherosclerosis enable doctors to truly "practice preventative medicine," Frossard says, but also the prescribed treatment will be more effective if the doctor knows "what genetic defect is causing the problem."

In separate research, Dr. Brian Robinson at St. George's Hospital in London found that a basic cell defect may be the cause of high blood pressure in about half of the people who develop it. He found that some people with high blood pressure had an abnormal reaction to calcium in their muscle cells. Robinson's research *(American Journal of Cardiology)* is still in the elementary stages but he hopes to be able to identify who has these cell defects and how their blood pressure can be properly regulated.

Race

Four times as many black Americans develop high blood pressure as white Americans. One of every four blacks has high blood pressure, compared to one of every six Americans overall, the National Heart, Lung and Blood Institute reports. Researchers are not sure what causes the difference, but high blood pressure is usually more severe in blacks, starts earlier and can lead to more severe complications, like premature strokes. High blood pressure and its related diseases are the major cause of death of blacks in the U.S., according to Max Feinman in *Live Longer*.

One theory that explains racial differences in rates of high blood pressure is that people with ancestors from the tropics where salt is often lacking and fluid loss from perspiration is high are more likely to have a "salt retention gene" than people whose ancestoral home was outside the tropics. This "salt retention" gene when it is present in any race causes the body to retain fluids and increase blood pressure.

Here are the estimated rates of prevalence of high blood pressure in blacks and whites, based on the final report of the 1984 Joint National Committee on Detection, Evaluation, and Treatment of High Blood Pressure.

High Blood Pressure Rates

Age	*White*	*Black*
65-74	63%	76%
55-64	51%	71%
45-54	39%	62%
35-44	21%	40%
25-34	13%	19%
18-24	9%	10%

Heredity is believed to be part of the reason for higher blood pressure in blacks, but high stress levels may also affect it, Max Feinman suggests. Because of our society's racial prejudices, Feinman feels that blacks are under increased amounts of stress which magnify the high blood pressure problem.

Since the traditional black diet is high in salt, diet may also be a factor. And several studies have shown that poor people of any race will suffer more severely because their blood pressure problems often go undiagnosed and untreated. Since a disproportionate number of blacks in America are poor, they may not have access to regular health care and health education.

Gender

Who do you think of when you picture someone with high blood pressure? Do you think of a middle-aged man who is climbing the corporate ladder while supporting a family? Most of us think of men as the main victims of high blood pressure, but more women have high blood pressure than men. Especially during life changes like pregnancy and menopause, women are at high risk for developing high blood pressure. During the reproductive years, birth control pills increase the risk for women (see chapter 7).

Age

Children and High Blood Pressure

Dr. Andrew G. Aronfy, a Fellow of the American Academy of Petiatrics (F.A.A.P.), writes:

"Until about 10 to 15 years ago, most pediatricians did not own a blood pressure cuff. In those days, the practice of pediatrics stopped at puberty, and blood pressure measurements were not part of a routine physical examination.

"During the past decade all that has changed. Other doctors started telling pediatricians that many young adults had high blood pressure, and they wondered when it started. When they asked pediatricians for blood pressure readings on their former patients, most pediatricians were embarrassed to confess that they had never checked it.

"Secondly, new discoveries about high blood pressure and coronary artery disease revealed that some cases may be strongly influenced by heredity. The tendency toward these diseases can be detected even in early childhood with high blood pressure readings and relatively simple blood tests, such as serum cholesterol and triglycerides. If a hereditary pattern seems to be developing, proper diet, exercise and lifestyle throughout the child's life may help reduce the inherited dangers.

"The most common cause of high blood pressure in children is kidney disease. A high blood pressure reading in a child may be a 'tip-off' that the child needs to be referred to an expert in nephrology to determine if kidney disease is present.

"There are other causes of high blood pressure in children. They are rare, and they are usually related to abnormal hormone production which may or may not be caused by a tumor.

"For all these reasons, all children should have

their blood pressure routinely checked from the time they are about 3 years old. If there is a history of high blood pressure or heart disease in the family, children should also have regular appropriate blood tests."

For accurate readings, children usually require a smaller blood pressure cuff. If you are monitoring your family's blood pressure at home, check with your doctor or public health nurse to see if you need a smaller cuff for your children.

If you suffer, or have suffered, from high blood pressure, be careful with your children's intake of salt, according to research published in the journal *Pediatrics*.

Craving for salt is acquired. Do not salt your children's food. Limit the amount of salt you use in food preparation. Limit the children's intake of highly salted foods like canned soups, potato chips, pickles and cured meats. If children do not grow up with salt, they will not crave it, and you will lower their risk of getting high blood pressure in the future.

The Elderly and High Blood Pressure

Authorities on heart and artery disease only recently began to acknowledge the unique aspects of high blood pressure in the older population and, as is often the case with such changes of direction in medicine, there is debate among medical leaders on how to treat the disorder.

The dimensions of the problem are not in dispute, however. According to William B. Abrams of Merck Sharp & Dohme Research Laboratories, more than half of the U.S. population over the age of 65 suffers from essential hypertension (high blood pressure not caused by some other condition such as kidney failure). "In the near future, this will translate into 10 to 25 million elderly people with high blood pressure who are at increased risk for congestive heart failure, strokes, heart attacks and certain types of aneurysms," he said.

"Not so long ago it was fashionable to ignore a little bit of high blood pressure in an elderly person," said Dr. W. McFate Smith, Professor of Epidemiology, University of California School of Public Health, Berkeley. "Limited data establishing the risk of elevated blood pressure in the age group over 65, particularly for women; concern over the presumed greater side effects of drugs in the elderly, and alterations in responsiveness to high blood pressure medications that occur with aging" were some of the rationalizations used, Smith explained.

Many authorities used to believe that high blood pressure was a physiological consequence of aging which was necessary to perfuse vital organs like the brain. Lowering blood pressure could be counterproductive, they argued. A more recent concern was that the quality of life— freedom from possible adverse effects of drug treatment — would be compromised by drug therapy.

In contrast to these views, scientific evidence suggested high blood pressure was a significant risk factor for the elderly, according to Dr. Smith.

"Systolic blood pressure has been shown to be a predictor of coronary heart disease mortality well into the ninth decade, and since considerable life expectancy remains for those who have survived to their senior years, it seems logical to attempt to reduce the risk and preserve independence and life expectancy by controlling blood pressure," he explained. Even a nominal rise in blood pressure in the elderly will lead to an a higher occurrence of strokes, according to a study recorded in *Geriatrics* (35:34).

It took some time for researchers to establish the benefits of effective therapy among the elderly. The early literature, which studied stroke survivors and attempted to evaluate the influence of hypertension on stroke recurrence, provided inconsistent and conflicting information on the value of therapy, Dr. Smith noted. However, he pointed out, well-controlled clinical trials published in the last decade without exception show a reduction in the risk of stroke and suggest reduction in death rates.

"Treatment should take into account the combined effects of aging and high blood pressure on the cardiovascular system and the kidneys," said Dr. Abrams, a researcher in the area of blood pressure and the elderly.

According to Dr. Abrams, the major age-related heart and artery changes are stiffening of the arterial system (hardening of the arteries) which can lead to a progressive rise in systolic blood pressure. This can result in thickening of the muscle in the wall of the left ventricle of the heart, a condition known as left ventricular hypertrophy, frequently seen in old age.

In the past, drugs seeking approval were studied in younger patients and the special effects they would have in elderly were not known until the drug had been approved and elderly people were using it in large numbers.

In recent years this practice has changed. Dr. Abrams has been collaborating with the U.S. Food and Drug Adminstration (F.D.A.), medical researchers, and pharmaceutical companies, to see that elderly patients are increasingly represented in clincial trials of new drugs.

New studies aimed specificially at the problems of the elderly are also being done. "The case for treating diastolic hypertension in elderly patients is strong. The case for treating isolated systolic hypertension is being investigated in the Systolic Hypertension in the Elderly Program," said Dr. Abrams, one of the program's researchers. "Until the data is available, we must exercise our clinical judgment in reaching decisions on the treatment of systolic high blood pressure in the elderly."

Conclusion

If you are in a high risk group, don't despair and accept high blood pressure as inevitable. Most cases of hypertension can be controlled through non-drug therapy or prescription drugs. "Even extremely high pressure can be controlled in nine of ten victims," the Virginia Department of Health reports.

We have written this book because we believe if you understand high blood pressure and if you take wise steps to control it, you can lead a healthy, happy life.

Chapter Three

How Is Blood Pressure Measured?

Blood pressure is usually taken with an arm pressure cuff, called a *sphygmomanometer*, which name comes from two Greek words that mean pulse measurement. Blood pressure is taken in two readings: for example, 120/80. The first number refers to *systolic* pressure or the pressure which is produced as the heart contracts to pump blood out into the body. The second number refers to *diastolic* pressure, or the pressure which remains in the blood vessels as the heart relaxes to allow for the flow of blood into its pumping chambers.

Blood pressure is measured in millimeters of mercury, abbreviated as *mm Hg*. Mercury is used as a standard because it is much heavier than blood or water (13.6 times heavier), and its rises and falls accurately show the rises and falls in our blood pressure. Mercury was first used to measure blood pressure by Jean Leonard-Marie Poiseuille in Paris in the 1800s, and it continues to be used for blood pressure measurement today.

When someone takes your blood pressure, a tightly fitting cuff is wrapped around your upper arm. Air is pumped into the cuff which stops the flow of blood in your arm. A stethoscope is placed on the arm. While the cuff is inflated, nothing is heard because the blood flow has been completely cut off. As a valve is turned and the air begins to escape from the cuff, the first pulse sound is heard through the stethoscope. The height of the mercury or the number on the gauge is noted when the first pulse is heard. This is the systolic level. As the air continues to be released from the cuff, the pulse sounds get stronger, then fade. The diastolic pressure is the number noted on the gauge or the column of mercury when the pulse begins to fade.

Electronic or digital gauges have replaced the traditional column of mercury in most new blood pressure measuring devices. Automatic blood pressure monitors, where a cuff is automatically inflated around your arm at regular intervals and the blood pressure noted, are also becoming popular. Automatic monitors, known as ambulatory monitors, can be worn throughout the day and provide accurate readouts for the doctor under different conditions, like your working, sleeping and resting blood pressure levels.

The most accurate way of measuring blood pressure is having a catheter inserted into an artery. The catheter's electronic signal is recorded and the blood pressure is measured. This is sometimes used in people with hardening of the arteries to get more precise readings. Since this is the most invasive method and since most external methods are reasonably accurate, it is not used often.

Recording the full range of blood pressure, including the systolic highs and the diastolic resting pressure, may be the next step in diagnosing high blood pressure. A new monitor being developed at the Technion-Israel Institute of Technology in Haifa, Israel, will eliminate the need for the arm cuff and stethoscope. The experimental monitor uses a small wristband that is more comfortable than a cuff, according to its developers. Also, the reading will be taken in just one second, compared to more than a minute needed for present monitoring. Sensors in the new monitor will give doctors a printout of "waves" of blood pressure, providing more information than current techniques.

A similiar method, which records the sounds of the blood pulsing through the veins in a continuous wave of blood pressure levels, is now being researched at the Cardiovascular Center of Cornell University Medical College. Rather than having only the high (systolic) and the low (diastolic) readings, the waves will show a continuous reading of all the blood pressure levels on a printed graph.

Researchers hope that the new wave monitors will be available for use by doctors, hospitals and emergency workers within the next few years.

What blood pressure levels are considered normal?

"Normal" blood pressure readings are based on average blood pressures for different age groups. Generally, blood pressures increase as people get older. Thus a pressure reading, for example, of 139/89 might be considered normal for someone over 50 but too high for a younger person. Regardless of age, blood pressure at or above 140/90 which is sustained for a long period of time is considered high and will damage the body.

If the lower (diastolic) number is between 90-104, the high blood pressure is considered mild. Moderate is from 105-114 and severe is anything above 115, according to the National Heart, Lung and Blood Institute. Severe high blood pressure, more than 250/115, calls for immediate attention and should be treated as an emergency.

Many people are told they have a "borderline" case of high blood pressure. Usually these people have levels that are at the high end of "normal" or in the "mild" classification (140-150 systolic or 90-104 diastolic). Most doctors will not prescribe drugs at this stage but will encourage lifestyle changes to lower the blood pressure naturally, before it causes damage to the vital organs.

Both numbers are used to evaluate blood pressure problems, although at one time physicians were only worried about the diastolic (second) number in the reading. The diastolic level is still considered the most important but both are evaluated. A new report shows that a systolic number of 160 or more doubles the risk of stroke or heart attack even if the diastolic number is within the normal range. Usually both numbers will rise if high blood pressure is present, but now if someone has a high reading in either their diastolic or systolic levels, they should be treated for high blood pressure, warns Boston University's William Kannel, M.D.

Remember that you should not diagnose yourself. Only a doctor will be able to interpret your blood pressure readings and decide what course you need to follow to achieve a normal level of blood pressure.

What about unusually low blood pressure readings?

Some people have low blood pressure which can cause unusual tiredness but doesn't damage the body like high blood pressure. People with low blood pressure tend to live longer than average.

Who should have their blood pressure taken?

Everyone, even children should be tested. It's a simple, safe test that can even be done in the home if your doctor agrees that this would be helpful. High blood pressure not only can be harmful by itself, but it also can be a symptom of other serious conditions, like heart disease or kidney disease.

How often should it be taken?

In people with normal blood pressure levels, blood pressure should be taken a minimum of once a year, but twice a year is preferable. People at highest risk, those with parents who have had high blood pressure, blacks and people who are overweight should have it checked every six months.

If you have high blood pressure and your doctor recommends diet, losing weight and exercise as the first steps in control, you should monitor your blood pressure at least once every two weeks.

If a prescription drug is prescribed, the doctor may want to monitor your blood pressure twice a week until the effects of the drug are known. If the drug provides a stable blood pressure, it may only need to be checked every few months.

Blacks of all ages and women taking birth control pills should have their blood pressure checked at least twice a year. The first time "the pill" is taken your blood pressure should be monitored every second month for the first six months.

Regular monitoring of your blood pressure can help lower it as much as relaxation techniques, SRI International scientists have discovered. They encourage people to become comfortable with monitoring their blood pressure at home and to do it regularly. The scientists think that regular monitoring lowers blood pressure because it reduces the stress of monitoring and increases the patient's understanding of his own problem.

Who should take your blood pressure?

Your doctor should be the person to check your blood pressure, but not everyone goes to a doctor regularly. Public health nurses, pharmacists, dentists or monitoring machines in a shopping mall are alternative ways to have your blood pressure checked. Many communities offer regular health fairs where you can get yours checked, and some hospitals provide this service at no cost. Who checks your blood pressure is not as important as having it checked accurately and regularly.

Some doctors are strongly opposed to using shopping mall monitoring machines because they feel that the machines are not always accurate. However, sometimes any reading is better than none at all. If a monitoring machine shows an unusual reading, and you get to your doctor for a checkup, the machine has provided a valuable service.

For many people on blood pressure medication, monitoring is often required twice a week. If these people can learn to take their blood pressure readings at home, they could save a lot of money in visits to the doctor, save time and actually provide their doctor with more readings.

Should it be taken at home?

In many cases, blood pressure readings are higher in the doctor's office than they are at home. Doctors at the New York Hospital - Cornell University Medical College compared home blood pressure monitoring to levels recorded in the doctor's office. "Home readings were lower and more accurate ... and reflect the overall level of BP more reliably than office readings," the doctors concluded in *Hypertension* (6:574-578).

Many doctors are now encouraging their patients with high blood pressure to monitor their own levels and record them at home. Patients bring their "blood pressure diary" to each checkup by the doctor. This way, the doctor can evaluate the blood pressure based on the normal daily blood pressure, rather than on an inflated blood pressure taken in a stressful visit to the doctor's office. Higher office readings have been refered to as "white coat hypertension" (*Journal of the American Medical Association* 247:992-996), because blood pressure sometimes rises when patients feel stressed by a visit to the doctor.

Taking your blood pressure at home can also provide the doctor with more information since more readings can be taken and because home readings are more convenient and less expensive. A report in the *British Medical Journal* (285:1691-1694) says that home blood pressures are as accurate as clinic readings, and, because they are recorded more frequently, they provide more useful information.

James Lynch, director of the Psychophysiological Clinic at the University of Maryland Medical School, urges all patients to take their blood pressure at home, at work, and during different stressful situations. All readings should be recorded with any unusual circumstances noted. Lynch finds that knowing their blood pressure levels helps people learn their own reactions to stress and what everyday activities increase their blood pressure.

Home monitoring itself can be a factor in lowering your blood pressure. A recent study in Seattle showed blood pressure levels lowered by 10 mm Hg. or more in 43 percent of people when they monitored their blood pressure at home. The researchers believe that regular monitoring fosters an increased awareness of blood pressure and helps the patient to remember that he has a serious problem. He then works harder to make lifestyle changes that will improve his health.

How do you take a blood pressure reading?

Anyone can learn to take blood pressure readings accurately. It is easier to have someone else take your reading, but even people living alone can take their readings at home with the right equipment and training.

First, we'll give you a detailed step-by-step approach to taking someone's blood pressure with a stethoscope and a sphygmomanometer with a standard gauge.

The first reading is the most accurate, so after you learn the technique you will always want to take the reading the first time. Once the cuff has been inflated around the arm and then a second reading is attempted, it won't be as accurate. If the first reading is not successful you should wait at least 30 minutes before trying again.

Sphygmomanometer and Stethoscope

1. Have the person who is having their blood pressure checked sit beside a table. (Let's call this person Jill). Let Jill relax for three to five minutes before taking the reading. Lay Jill's right arm so the lower part of the arm is resting comfortably on the table. The palm of her hand should be face up and her elbow slightly bent.

2. Take the cuff of the sphygmomanometer and wrap it on the upper arm, directly above where the arm bends (opposite the elbow) on Jill's right arm. The tubes that come out of the cuff and are attached to the gauge should be right on the center of the arm just above the bent elbow. Some cuffs have an arrow to show where the center of the cuff is so it can be directly over the center of the arm. Wrap the cuff around the arm so it is snug. It should not be too tight or too loose. It should be about half an inch above the bend in the arm. Do not get any clothes under the cuff or they could affect the reading.

3. Place the stethoscope around your neck. The ends of the stethoscope do not join together as a

circle, but are bent. When the stethoscope is placed in your ears, the ends should be pointing towards your eyes. Make sure that you place the stethoscope around your neck so the ends will be in the right direction.

4. Position yourself so that you can easily see the gauge where you will have to read the blood pressure levels.

5. With your index finger, find the pulse spot in Jill's arm. By pressing gently underneath the cuff, right above the elbow, you should be able to find her artery and her pulse. Some people's pulse point is off center, so it is important to find it first with your index finger.

6. Once you have found the pulse, place the stethoscope underneath the cuff and directly on that pulse spot. Put the ends of the stethoscope in your ears. Keep one hand pressing the stethoscope firmly on the pulse spot throughout the reading. You will not hear the pulse until you start taking the reading.

7. With your other hand, grasp the bulb used to inflate the cuff. Tighten the screw valve leading to the bulb. Hold the bulb so that you will be able to slowly loosen the valve, while holding the bulb in the same hand, after the cuff has been inflated.

8. Start squeezing the bulb. Watch the level on the gauge. For someone with a history of normal blood pressure inflate the cuff until the level reaches 200. For someone with a history of high blood pressure, inflate the cuff to 220 or 240. You should pump it at least 30 points higher than the normal systolic (or first) reading for that person. You want to pump it up high enough the first time so a second reading doesn't have to be taken.

9. Loosen the screw valve just a little, so the level falls very slowly. Once you get used to taking blood pressure, you can allow the pressure to drop quickly, but in the beginning, you will need the reading to be as slow as possible to be most accurate.

10. As soon as you hear the pulse, note the number on the gauge. This is the systolic or first reading.

11. Keep your eye on the gauge and remember the number where the pulse fades away or changes to a muffled sound. In some people it is normal to have a beat continue to zero, so you need to train yourself to listen to the change in the pulse. This second reading is the diastolic pressure.

12. Loosen the screw completely so the cuff finishes deflating.

13. Remove the stethoscope from your ears.

14. Remove the cuff from Jill's arm.

15. Write down the two readings, in the order that they were taken. The higher number will be first and the lower number second. The reading should be written like a division problem, for example 120/80. When speaking about the reading you would say, "Jill's blood pressure is 120 over 80."

Other Sphygmomanometers

Using a standard sphygmomanometer and stethoscope is fine for taking someone else's blood pressure, but it is difficult to take your own this way (although it can be done). The easiest way to take your own blood pressure is to purchase a sphygmomanometer with a built-in stethoscope. Most of these models will provide a digital readout of your blood pressure. All you need to learn is to place the cuff and the built-in stethoscope in the right place and inflate the cuff.

Any model you purchase should come with instructions on how to use it and how to care for it. For example, the bulb that is used to inflate the cuff can develop holes and blisters if it is left in direct heat or sunlight. Follow your manufacturer's directions for the best care of your sphygmomanometer.

Once you understand the basic principles of how to take blood pressure, you can decide which type of blood pressure monitoring equipment would be best for you. If your doctor wants you to monitor your blood pressure at home, he or she may prescribe a sphygmomanometer so your insurance will help cover the cost. More expensive models are not necessarily more accurate than cheaper models, although more expensive brands are usually made for frequent use by many people.

How can you be sure that your technique is correct?

After you practice taking someone's blood pressure, you should take your sphygmomanometer to your doctor or nurse and have them observe you taking a blood pressure reading. Your doctor will be able to offer tips to improve your technique and accuracy and you will both feel more secure about the readings you obtain at home. Have your sphygmomanometer checked to make sure it is accurate compared with the office sphygmomanometers.

What can cause an inaccurate reading?

Great stress, physical exercise, and the time of day can all affect your blood pressure levels. Don't smoke just before checking your blood pressure because smoking can cause a higher reading. Don't walk up stairs or walk briskly to your doctor's appointment. It is best to have been calm and relaxed in a resting position for about five minutes before your blood pressure is taken.

Your position during a blood pressure reading is very important. If you raise your arm when your blood pressure is taken, the level will often be lower than if you let your arm hang down at your side. If you stand it will be different than if you are sitting or lying down. The most accurate way to measure blood pressure is to sit down with your arm resting on a table level with your heart.

Most times, blood pressure is measured in your right arm. However, blocked arteries or other problems in your arm may cause inaccurate blood pressure readings. The first time your blood pressure is measured, it should be taken in both arms and both readings should be recorded, including the arm that was used. Then, if the readings are similiar, the right arm can be used for future monitoring.

A woman who has had a mastectomy or someone who has had a limb amputated should not have her blood pressure taken on that side of their body.

If the stethoscope is pressed into the arm with too much force the diastolic blood pressure reading can be as much as ten percent too high, reveals the *Western Journal of Medicine* (141: 193). The stethoscope needs to be pressed against the artery with firm, but gentle, pressure, the article warns, or you may be needlessly treated for high blood pressure.

Overweight people or people who are very tiny, like children, may need a different cuff than the standard size. A regular cuff is usually between 4 3/4 and 5 inches wide. An overweight person would need an obese cuff which is over 6 inches wide. And children should use a narrow cuff or their readings will be lower than their true blood pressure level.

You can copy the chart in the back of this book to help record your blood pressure readings. If you are taking prescription drugs of any kind, be sure to note those with your blood pressure readings.

What is false high blood pressure?

Many people diagnosed as having high blood pressure are wrongly diagnosed. Researchers in Canada found that "one of every four people who appeared to have high blood pressure actually did not," according to Prevention magazine.

Dr. Nicholas Birkett, the study's chief researcher, speculates that those people experienced "white-coat apprehension" — nervousness at being in the presence of a doctor or nurse. This caused their blood pressure to be unusually high during the doctor's office reading.

When blood pressure was taken twice more on two separate occasions, the people were found to have normal blood pressure.

Dr. Birkett's finding has been confirmed by investigators at New York Hospital - Cornell University Medical Center (*Journal of the American Medical Association* 259: 225-228). They compared blood pressure measurements obtained by doctors with readings taken by an automatic arm recorder worn during the day. For both hypertensive patients and those with normal blood pressure, the highest blood pressure recorded was the one taken by the physician.

Blood pressure levels taken by a technician were lower, and the levels recorded on the automatic recorder worn at home were even lower.

Women are most likely to be misdiagnosed as having high blood pressure when their levels are taken by a male physician, the Cornell study shows. Levels are more accurate when taken by a technician, although the researchers aren't sure why. Thomas G. Pickering, M.D., one of the researchers, suggests that the doctor is seen as more of an authority figure and causes more anxiety than a technician. They conclude that many women, especially younger women, who are classed as having high blood pressure are misdiagnosed — they really have normal levels. Having a woman doctor or technician take the reading can give a more accurate level.

Lawrence Krakoff, M.D., of the Mount Sinai Medical Center in New York, often uses ambulatory monitors which can be worn throughout the day to provide accurate readouts under different conditions, like working, sleeping and resting. Fifty percent of his patients with mild high blood pressure have lower diastolic levels when an ambulatory monitor is used, Dr. Krakoff explains.

Hardening of the arteries in the elderly may also

cause high, inaccurate blood pressure readings, according to Dr. Frank H. Messerli, a blood pressure specialist, who was quoted in the *New England Journal of Medicine* (312:1548-51).

Dr. Messerli discovered that people over 65 with hardened arteries had higher blood pressure when monitored with a blood pressure cuff than their true blood pressure taken using a needle inside the arteries.

For an accurate diagnosis of mild high blood pressure, Dr. Birkett recommends taking three or four separate readings over as long as six months. Home blood pressure readings, or 24-hour monitoring, can help give doctors a better picture of a patient's true blood pressure.

Chapter Four

How Serious Is High Blood Pressure?

High blood pressure contributes, directly or indirectly, to about one million deaths a year. Compared to people with normal blood pressure, people with uncontrolled high blood pressure have:

—seven times as many strokes

—four times as much congestive heart failure

—three times as much coronary heart disease.

Heart attacks, the largest single cause of death in the U.S., account for 36 percent of all deaths among males aged 35 to 64. Each year, over 125,000 employed persons die of high-blood-pressure-related cardiovascular (heart and artery) disease.

The economic costs of cardiovascular disease are staggering: $26 billion each year in direct costs and $54 billion in indirect costs, Knoll Pharmaceuticals estimates. Each year over 29 million work days are lost due to high blood pressure related illnesses. This translates into lost earnings of $1.5 billion.

High blood pressure is a major risk factor associated with development of cardiovascular disease. Just as too much air pressure can damage the lining and surface of automobile tires, persistent high blood pressure can damage the interior and exterior of human arteries. It can also damage key organs, such as the brain, heart, kidneys and eyes. High blood pressure can also cause additional strain on the body and cause weak body parts to fail.

Strokes

Strokes are the third leading cause of death in the United States. People with high blood pressure, people with a family or personal history of heart disease or strokes, diabetics, smokers, blacks, women taking oral contraceptives, men and those over age 60 are at the highest risk of having a stroke. People with high blood pressure have seven times as many strokes as people with normal blood pressure.

Controlling high blood pressure can reduce your risk of stroke, researchers at the Mayo Clinic reported in the *Journal of the American Medical Association*

(258: 214-217). They found that "as control of high blood pressure increased the stroke rates decreased." In the study, "controlled" blood pressure referred to levels below 95 mm Hg. diastolic. It did not matter if the blood pressure was controlled through prescription drugs or natural methods as long as it was below 95.

A stroke occurs when blood vessels become blocked and cut off the flow of blood to the brain, or when blood vessels break and allow blood to leak into brain tissue. If the brain is deprived of blood, the brain cells die and cannot be replaced. Permanent damage or death can occur. It may take years for high blood pressure to weaken and damage blood vessels, but a stroke can happen within seconds with no warning. A stroke can last for just a few minutes or it can last for hours.

If the right part of the brain is damaged by a stroke, the person could be paralyzed on the left side and experience a loss in perception, spacing and memory. If the left part of the brain is damaged, the victim could be paralyzed on the right side and have difficulty with speech and remembering words.

If you are at high risk for stroke, you should learn the early warning signs and be prepared to act on them. Here are some of the signs of a small stroke, as identified by the American Heart Association. Report all early warning signs of stroke to your doctor immediately. If a stroke is caught in the early stages, you may prevent a fatality:

> change in vision, like a flash of blindness or double vision
> difficulty with speech
> unexplained headaches or dizziness
> impaired judgment
> numbness, weakness or tingling sensations
> sudden change in mental abilities
> sudden change in personality
> any symptoms that seem to occur only on one side of the body.

However, you can reduce your risk of having a stroke if you lower high blood pressure, control diabetes, quit smoking or using tobacco, lose weight and begin a healthy low-fat, low-salt diet.

Coronary Artery Disease

Coronary artery disease kills more people in our society than any other illness. What causes it? "Uncontrolled high blood pressure is the biggest risk factor in coronary artery disease," explains Sandy Sorrentino, Ph.D., author of *Coping With High Blood Pressure*.

The disease begins when fatty streaks form in the inner linings of the coronary arteries, the arteries which feed blood to the heart muscle. Autopsies show that fatty streaks can begin in the main artery of the body, the aorta, in infancy. These buildups are frequently found in the smaller coronary arteries by the time children become teenagers.

The fatty streaks may build into atheromas, which are small raised plaques of mushy cholesterol, fat and "foam cells" on the inner walls of the arteries. As the plaques grow, they may start to come together and seriously constrict the flow of blood within the arteries. Scar tissue may begin to grow under the fatty plaque, and this scar tissue may become "hardened" by deposits of calcium. This hardening of the arteries is called atherosclerosis. At this point the arteries have reached an advanced state of disease, and the flow of blood may be severely constricted by hard, chalky plaque, which may not regress or shrink even with the best of care.

High blood pressure speeds the development of atherosclerosis, and the hardened arteries in turn increase the blood pressure, so a vicious cycle is developed. Also, high cholesterol levels, smoking and being overweight are all causes of high blood pressure and atherosclerosis.

Atherosclerosis is also a major cause in heart attacks and heart problems. Heart attacks may happen after a piece of an atherosclerotic plaque comes loose and plugs a coronary artery or after a partial blockage from atherosclerosis upsets the rhythm of the heartbeat. During a heart attack, the heart may suddenly stop pumping blood effectively or go into a series of ineffective, twitching contractions called fibrillation. Fibrillation often can be stopped by an electrical shock given through the wall of the chest by an electronic defibrillator. After defibillation, the heart may recover its normal beat.

The survival of a heart attack victim depends upon the severity of the attack and upon the swiftness of medical attention. Coronary intensive care units in major hospitals are well-equipped to handle heart attack emergencies, and a quick ride in a ambulance to the hospital has saved many a life.

Knowing the warning signs of a heart attack may save your life, especially if you do not delay in seeking medical help. Some heart attacks are called silent heart attacks because there is no advance warning. However, many heart attacks are not unexpected because the victim has suffered, perhaps for years, from *angina pectoris* or pain in the chest. If a heart attack is not occurring, angina usually will go away after a few minutes of rest or after the administration of doctor-prescribed nitroglycerin, which is taken to dilate or expand the coronary arteries. Since people with high blood pressure are at increased risk for having a heart attack, be sure you know the symptoms:

> heavy pressure or a choking or squeezing sensation in the center of the chest

> chest pain which may radiate down one or both arms, across the back, or up the neck

> shortness of breath

> an unexplained sensation or feeling of fear

> perspiration

> nausea

> dizziness or lightheadedness

> weakness or a fainting sensation

> angina pain that lasts for more than a few minutes or that doesn't go away upon administratrion of nitroglycerin and rest.

All of these symptoms need not be present to

indicate that a heart attack is taking place. Some can be caused by other problems, like indigestion.

Congestive Heart Failure

High blood pressure can also place an extra burden on the heart, which in time will cause the heart to weaken. Fluid builds up in the body's tissues, and the kidneys may fail. Congestive heart failure occurs when fluid builds up around the heart and chokes it.

Kidney Problems

Uremia, caused by the progressive narrowing of the kidney blood vessels, can be caused by uncontrolled high blood pressure. The high blood pressure causes the arteries to become tighter and more narrow, which eventually reduces the blood pressure to the kidneys. The malfunctioning kidney responds by trying to increase the blood pressure, creating more problems.

Once the kidneys begin to function below normal, waste products like salt are not properly excreted. With salt and other normally excreted products remaining in the kidney, it continues to malfunction.

When the kidneys become damaged, they cannot be repaired. Kidney dialysis or a transplant can be used to solve the problem, but sudden death due to kidney failure could also occur.

Controlling blood pressure can prevent irreparable damage to your kidneys.

Brain Damage

Serious swelling of the brain can occur with uncontrolled high blood pressure. A person with a long history of uncontrolled high blood pressure or someone who experiences unusually high blood pressure is at highest risk. Brain damage or death could occur if the swelling is not treated immediately.

Loss of Vision

Just like blood vessels in the brain and throughout the body, high blood pressure also forces the small blood vessels in the eye to narrow. The capillaries in the eyes may begin to deteriorate due to lack of blood and a loss of vision, sometimes called "tunnel vision," or blindness can result.

The relationship between uncontrolled high blood

pressure and loss of vision has only recently been verified. Doctors are now aware of the importance of regular eye checkups as well as the monitoring of blood pressure levels when treating people with elevated blood pressure.

Higher Death Rates in Cancer Patients

High blood pressure has been associated with higher death rates in cancer patients (Journal of the National Cancer Institute 77:1,63). The higher the blood pressure, the more likely the patient was to die from the cancer, the researchers discovered.

Conclusion

As we write this book we are reminded of how interrelated many diseases are. We cannot isolate one disease, like high blood pressure, and treat only that. We must consider the condition of the body as a whole.

In the same way, we must consider the well-being of our bodies as a whole. The health factors we will give you in Part Two of this book are not just to control your high blood pressure. They will also help your heart, your kidneys, and your over-all health.

Part Two

Lowering Blood Pressure Naturally

You know from Part One of this book that high blood pressure is a serious condition that must not be ignored. You also know that some of its causes may be out of your control — like heredity or race or gender.

However, the reason we are writing this book is that there are far many more factors that you can control about high blood pressure. No one should wring his hands in despair because he is at higher risk, and no one should become complacent because he is at lower risk. How you live your life — your eating habits, your lifestyle, your values — have far more to do with your health than you imagine.

These natural causes and effects on high blood pressure are what Part Two of this book is about.

Here's information about natural ways to either avoid or deal with high blood pressure.

If you want to grow beautiful flowers, you must provide them with good nutrients, healthy growing conditions, and you must go to the trouble of pulling out harmful weeds that might choke their growth. In the same way, if you want to enjoy beautiful health, you must nuture and care for your body. In Part Two we will discuss nutrients you need, habits to help you, and we will point out "weeds" that may be choking your well-being. It is our goal to help you control your blood pressure as much as you can by natural ways.

High blood pressure *can* be lowered without drugs. For example, in one recent university test, 85.31 percent of patients with high blood pressure were able to quit taking their medication. Even without drugs, their blood pressures remained lower than when they were on drugs. The hundreds of people in the study also found that their blood cholesterol levels dropped 26 percent. The doctor in charge of the program said, "You lose your tiredness. You feel much more active. You have a general feeling of well being." The patients learned some of the health secrets we will describe and began making changes in their eating, exercise habits and lifestyle.

If you have high blood pressure be sure to carefully consult with your physician before discontinuing medication or treating the condition yourself.

Chapter Five

Dietary Factors in Lowering Blood Pressure

This chapter will focus on the foods we eat and how they affect blood pressure. The dietary guidelines we recommend are much like those used by the Pritikin Longevity Centers in the United States. Not long ago, a research team from Loma Linda University studied the results of the Pritikin program, which also included moderate daily exercise such as walking.

Overweight patients lost an average of more than ten pounds. Eighty-five percent of the patients who were taking high blood pressure drugs were able to quit taking these drugs, with their doctors' permission because their blood pressures had dropped to acceptable levels.

Cholesterol levels dropped 26 percent. Many

people who had been taking drugs to control their blood cholesterol were able to stop taking medicine. The level of other blood fats also dropped nearly 26 percent. Forty percent of the patients who were diabetics were able, under medical supervision, to stop taking insulin. The patients became more mentally alert and performed better on tests of mental ability. Many patients lost their tiredness and required much less sleep.

This type of diet tries to work against high blood pressure in 3 ways:

1) it is low in calories so people can lose weight,

2) it is low in sodium to help sodium-sensitive people,

3) it is low in cholesterol to help limit damage on the heart and arteries caused by high blood pressure.

Before Changing Your Eating Habits

Evaluate your present eating habits. Note how many high-sodium, high-calorie and high-cholesterol foods you eat on a daily basis. Look for ways to improve your diet and make a commitment to yourself that you will try to improve your health through your diet.

Consider the effects dietary changes may have on your body. Also, consider the effects a drastic change in eating habits may have on your mind and emotions.

First, don't overdose on fiber. Your body has had years to adjust to the lack of fiber in the typical American diet and it may take a few days or weeks to become adjusted to higher levels of fiber.

If you have a problem with too frequent elimination or flatulence, cut back a little on high-fiber foods like bran muffins and bran bread. Substitute foods which contain adequate but lighter fiber, like oatmeal, brown rice or bread made with half whole wheat flour and half unbleached white flour. Each person is unique, so you may have to experiment to find out how much fiber is right for you.

Secondly, if a total change in eating habits is too hard, gradually change your habits by substituting whole grain cereals for bacon or sausage at breakfast, making sandwiches with whole wheat bread, or pulling the fat-laden skin and breading off of deep fat fried chicken. Many people can move in little steps toward a much more healthy diet.

Your approach to eating the foods that are best for your health needs to be continued throughout your life. By slowly making changes, you may be able to live with them for a longer time. Sometimes, drastic changes in diet are too difficult, and the person completely reverts back to his old eating habits.

Learning what foods are beneficial and what foods should be avoided is the first step. If you are only able to follow the following dietary recommendations in half of the foods you eat, you will still receive a substantial benefit. The more that the recommendations are followed, the greater will be the benefits. Even one step in the right direction will be helpful in improving your total health.

At home or in a restaurant, try to eat foods that are lightly cooked: broiled, steamed, roasted or baked in their own juices. Raw fruit and vegetables are often the best selection.

Drink enough water each day to produce a quart of light colored urine. Water is necessary for regular bowel movements, to help prevent kidney stones, to protect us from disease and to prevent dehydration. Drinking "hard" certified pure spring water is recommended. Coauthor Frank Cawood prefers Mountain Valley Water. He says, "It's low in sodium and has a good balance of necessary minerals like calcium and magnesium."

Also, older people need to be especially careful to drink enough water each day, because many elderly people lose their sense of thirst, reports a recent study in the *New England Journal of Medicine*. Since they may not feel thirsty or uncomfortable, older people can become dehydrated.

Foods That Are Good For You

As a general guide, here is a list of foods that are good for you because they are low in salt, fat, and cholesterol.

lean veal
skimmed milk
yogurt (low fat)
skimmed milk cheeses
peppers
dried beans
dried peas
whole wheat noodles
lean beef
olive oil
onions
vinegar
dried rice
dried barley
chicken (with skin removed)
fish (not canned in oil)
baked potatoes (with little or no butter or margarine)
homemade whole grain yeast bread (made

without salt or baking powder)
natural cereals (without salt added)
beverages which don't contain fat or caffeine
fresh fruits and vegetables
cottage cheese (low fat or dry curd varieties)

Foods To Avoid

Here are some foods and preparations to avoid as you seek to lower your blood pressure naturally.

canned soup
pickles or olives
potato chips or pretzels
french fries
canned vegetables
canned meats
smoked meat or fish
luncheon meat
salt cured ham
pork
sausage
pepperoni
hot dogs
instant cocoa mixes
bacon
cheese
salted nuts
most crackers
sauerkraut
liver
shrimp
lobster
herring
sardines
caviar
anchovies
flavored gelatin
pizza

most processed food
"fast food"
most frozen dinners
beer
tomato sauce
most sauces
gravy
boullion
ketchup
mustard
relish
horseradish
chili sauce
steak sauce
Worcestershire sauce
soy sauce
peanut butter

chocolate milk
ice cream
milk shakes
baking powder
baking soda
garlic salt
onion salt
celery salt
salad dressings
cake mixes
pancakes mixes
muffin mixes
pudding mixes
biscuit mixes
cornbread mixes
many laxatives
meat tenderizer

MSG (monosodium glutamate)
foods containing sodium bicarbonate
foods containing disodium phosphate
salted butter or salted margarine

The rest of the chapter will elaborate on some of the key dietary factors which affect blood pressure.

Salt : Good and Bad News

You may be already preparing yourself to hear that one more flavor you love — salt — is bad for your health. Is there nothing you can enjoy eating anymore?

Salt itself isn't bad for your health. You may remember how your grandparents used salt liberally to cure and preserve meats in the smokehouse on their farm — and no one mentioned high blood pressure back then. And you may know that in the Bible Jesus says, "Ye are the salt of the earth," indicating that even thousands of years ago salt was a valuable commodity for preserving food and stimulating taste buds. The word from which we get our word "salary" comes from the Latin word "sal," meaning salt. Roman soldiers were sometimes said to be "worth their salt" because they were often paid in salt rather than actual money.

Why, then, all the fuss about removing salt from our diets? Why is it so bad all of a sudden? Is this a passing medical "fad"?

Unfortunately the answer is "no" — this is not a passing problem. What has happened is that we have simply "overdosed" on a good thing to the point that it has become a bad thing.

Salt, or sodium chloride, is essential to life. It is an important mineral in the body. Without it we would die. Salt maintains fluid levels between the cells and the blood system and acts as an electrolyte to help chemical and electrical reactions in the body.

However, our bodies are equipped to handle only so much salt. Dr. Cleaves M. Bennett, author of *Control Your High Blood Pressure Without Drugs*, says, "The quantities of salt we actually eat are a great burden on our systems. It's so destructive. As we eat more salt than the kidneys can readily excrete, over a long period of time, many years, salt builds up in the body .... The body's way to get rid of more of that salt... is to push it out through the kidneys by raising the blood pressure" (p. 36-37).

The average American eats five to 10 grams of sodium, or one-third to one-fifth of an ounce of salt per day. This is much more salt than is needed for bodily functions. Most people only need one-tenth that amount. Recent studies indicate that some people need as little as one-fifth of a gram (200 milligrams) of salt per day. However, there are exceptions. Hard labor, profuse sweating, pregnancy, and breast feeding may increase the need for salt up to two grams per day.

Most people will question whether they really consume one-third to one-fifth of an ounce of salt per day, but processed foods that North Americans eat are usually filled with salt. Any food that comes in a can, a frozen package or a box is likely to have salt added as a preservative or flavor enhancer.

Table salt and salty products can be easy to avoid, but it is this "hidden salt" that often has consumers stumped. The Food and Drug Administration (FDA) is now requiring soft-drink manufacturers to list the sodium content of their drinks on the bottles or cans. Many products are required to list their sodium content, but be wary of their advertising and labeling. Low sodium can mean different things for different foods. For example, sodium-free drinks have to contain less than five milligrams (mg.) of salt per 12 oz. can. "Very low sodium" will be less than 35 mg. per can and "low sodium" can be placed on cans containing 140 mg. of salt or less according to the FDA's standards.

A typical slice of bread may contain over 200 milligrams (mg.) of salt, a bowl of corn flakes over 300 mg., a bowl of canned soup over 1000 mg., a TV dinner over 2500 mg., a chicken dinner from a fast food restaurant over 2000 mg., and a large dill pickle over 1000 mg.

Studies of different nations around the world show that high blood pressure is a problem only in societies where people eat a lot of sodium, usually in the form of salt. (Sodium, part of the sodium chloride salt molecule, is also found in other forms. Technically, it is the sodium in salt which is the villian in our fight against high blood pressure. In this book, we will continue to use "salt" as a more common term.)

High blood pressure rates are in direct proportion to the amount of salt consumed. The more salt that a particular society consumes, the greater the number of cases of severe high blood pressure. It is significant that the Greenland Eskimos and the Amazon Indians, who eat very little salt have very little high blood pressure. But in the north of Japan, high blood pressure is common among the people whose diet contains large amounts of salt. Of course, in such societies other factors may also be at work, but the strong relationship between salt consumption and high blood pressure should be noted.

Perhaps you feel that you are just a "salt lover" because foods don't taste right to you without salt. But scientific studies indicate that salt preference is a learned habit—an acquired taste. As people reduce the amount of salt in their diets, they experience new flavor sensations that were masked by the large amounts of salt they used to eat. The true flavor of vegetables can be hidden by cooking with too much salt. In this sense, excessive salt can be a taste destroyer rather than a flavor enhancer.

One scientific study on salt consumption deals with twins. One twin was put on a low-salt diet. The other twin continued to consume a diet high in salt. After a few weeks, the twin on the low-salt diet learned to consume less salt and prefered to eat less salt. The other twin still was in the habit of consuming more salt and continued to prefer the high salt diet.

It will take about three months to lose the craving for salt, according to Mrs. Dash, a producer of no-salt products.

If you are concerned about giving up flavor in your cooking, a little creativity can help add "spice" to your food while lowering the salt content. You do not have to sacrifice flavor when you cut down on sodium if you follow these suggestions from *Prevention* magazine and other authorities:

> Remove the salt shaker from your table.

> Never use salt in cooking or reduce your use of salt in recipes by at least one half.

> Use lemon juice on food instead instead of salt.

> Don't use onion or garlic salt as spices as they are just "flavored" salt. Use real onion or garlic for more flavor without the salt.

> When baking cakes, cookies, pies and puddings, use extracts instead of salt and reduce the sugar.

> Avoid store bought mixes for puddings, cakes, muffins, biscuits, cornbread, pancakes, etc. If you prepare your own from scratch you can control your ingredients.

> Read all labels to determine the sodium content and buy low sodium products whenever possible. Watch for any additives that contain the word sodium, like sodium chloride, sodium hydroxide, monosodium glutamate (MSG), sodium bicarbonate, disodium phosphate, sodium benzoate, sodium propionate, sodium saccharin, disodium sulfite or others that contain salt like baking soda, baking powder and brine. Avoid these.

> Learn about the many natural herbs, spices, and fruit peels that are available. You may decide to grow your own or to experiment with store-bought

herbs.

> Use one of several salt-free mixtures of herbs and spices that are available for seasonings.

> Enjoy Mexican, Cajun, and Tex-Mex foods. The strong spices give flavor without adding salt. Beware of oriental food — it can be high in MSG which is high in salt.

> To spice chicken dishes, add fruit such as mandarin oranges or pineapples.

> Marinate chicken, fish, beef or poultry in orange juice or lemon juice. Add a homemade mustard or honey glaze.

> Marinate meat in wine or add wine to sauces or soups. If you thoroughly cook the dish, the alcohol will evaporate but the flavor will be enhanced.

> Use fresh vegetables whenever possible. However, if you must used canned vegetables, wash them in cool water before using. Rinsing will help remove some of the salt added in the canning process.

> Just a little green pepper, parsley, paprika or red pepper can add a lot of flavor to a meal.

> Be sure to keep the meals attractive and in clude a variety of colors and textures. Most people are more tempted to add salt when the meal appears bland.

> Avoid taking sodium ascorbate, a formulation of vitamin C that contains sodium. If you need a vitamin C supplement while cutting back on sodium, ascorbic acid or calcium ascorbate forms of vitamin C are acceptable.

> Drink water with your meals and avoid soft drinks. Soft drinks are high in sugar which dulls your taste buds and makes it more difficult to give up salt. Also, many carbonated drinks are high in salt content. Even some sugar free soft drinks contain salt as sodium saccharin.

A test to show how much salt you are really consuming is available and may help some people monitor or reduce their sodium intake, says a study in *Archives of Internal Medicine* (144:1963-5). Thirty percent of people in the study had lower salt intake when they were using a chloride titrator strip at home. If you are not sure of your current salt intake or if you want to monitor your diet, check with your doctor about the titrator strip test.

Many scientific studies show that reducing salt intake will lower blood pressure in most people by a significant amount. Getting salt intake down into the range of 500 mg. of salt per day helps the most. Reducing salt intake lowers blood pressure dramatically in some people because they have a hereditary tendency to hold on to salt or sodium. Thus, the benefits of reduced salt consumption are greatest for some of the people who need the benefits the most.

Certain people seem to be "salt retentive", and others are not as affected by salt, according to studies by Dr. L. K. Dahl in *Circulation Research* (40: 1131-4). He found that some animals will develop high blood pressure, no matter how much salt they ingest. However, some people can consume large quantities of salt and never develop high blood pressure. Since there are not any tests to show who is salt retentive and who is not (although some are in the development stages), health professionals recommend that everyone reduce their salt intake as part of their high blood pressure treatment.

We believe so strongly in the importance of lowering salt consumption that we have prepared a series of 14 daily menu plans to help you choose to eat correctly. They are found in Appendix Two, page 205. We also have compiled many delicious recipes for low-salt, low-fat and high fiber dishes that you can enjoy and these are found in Appendix Three, page 219. Please take the crucial step of caring enough about yourself and your family's health that you will get control over this potential villain, salt.

Diets Low In Fiber

Fiber supplements were given to people in one recent study, reported by Danish researchers in the *Lancet* 2(8559):622-3. The people in the study discovered that their systolic pressure (the upper number) dropped an average of ten points and the diastolic pressure dropped an average of five points in just three months. However, people in the study who took a placebo (a harmless, fake supplement) did not experience a change in their blood pressure.

Low-fiber diets have also been linked to heart and artery disease, constipation, appendicitis, diverticulosis, cancer of the large bowel, colon cancer, hemorrhoids and obesity.

One hundred years ago, the diet of the American and Canadian people contained an adequate amount of natural food fiber. Most bread was made with whole wheat flour which contained bran, the outer fibrous part of the wheat kernel. Coronary heart disease was rare at this time, and few people were troubled with appendicitis, diverticulosis, cancer of the large bowel, constipation, hemorrhoids, obesity or high blood pressure.

Then, in the last quarter of the 19th century,

American industry made two discoveries which were hailed as breakthroughs. The first invention was the development of high speed steel roller mills for flour milling. Food companies could produce a fine white flour which tasted better than most whole wheat flour and was less likely to spoil. The second development was the growth of the canning industry, and the canning process greatly reduced food fiber content.

These two changes took place over several years, and no one noticed that anything was wrong. But in the 20th century, scientists became puzzled at the persistent rise in certain death rates and obesity. Commentators noticed that people in less developed countries didn't suffer very much from these ills.

In the 1940s and 50s, Dr. Denis Burkitt, a British surgeon, noticed that he never found a case of diverticular disease or cancer of the colon in the thousands of rural tribesmen of East Africa that were autopsied. Further research showed that obesity, appendicitis, heart attacks, constipation and hemorrhoids were also extremely rare. Dr. Burkitt thought that the amount of fiber in the diet was the key. He, and other doctors like Cleave, Trowell and Heaton, investigated what happened to tribes who moved to African cities and adopted a typical, low-fiber western diet.

The results confirmed the hypothesis. On a diet that had been depleted of bran and other fiber, many Africans became obese and developed all the other ills of western civilization (*Journal of the American Medical Association* 229: 1068-74). Dr. Burkitt also linked high blood pressure with a lack of fiber in the diet (*JR College of Physicians* 9:138-46).

Diets High In Fat

Americans now consume almost 40 percent of their total calories from fat. High-fat diets along with other factors can cause hardening of the arteries which leads to higher and higher blood pressure over the years. Low-fat diets are associated with low blood pressure. Cutting fat intake levels in half can have a dramatic effect in reducing many cases of high blood pressure. A recent study by the U.S. Department of Agriculture found that eating less saturated fat could bring blood pressure down even in the absence of taking other beneficial measures. One researcher connected with the study said that it produced strong evidence that high fat diets are undesirable because they lead to high blood pressure as well as other problems.

Educating yourself to identify and avoid high fat foods, as well as increasing your fiber intake are two of the most important steps you can take in changing to a healthier diet.

It is important to learn that all fats are not the same. *Saturated fats* raise the blood cholesterol and trigylceride levels. They are primarily found in animal and dairy products such as fats in meats, egg yolks, milk, butter, cheese, cream and a few vegetable fats, such as coconut oil and hydrogenated vegetable shortenings. Saturated fats are generally hard or solid at room temperature.

Replacing saturated fats with unsaturated fats, especially olive oil or fish oil may also help reduce high blood pressure. Remember, fats are present not only in meat and dairy products but also in fried foods, chips, creamed sauces, mayonnaise and pastries to name a few. Learn to read labels on cans and packages, looking for the fat content listed.

Polyunsaturated fats help to lower the levels of cholesterol in the blood and reduce the risk of high blood pressure. They are mostly derived from plant and vegetable sources, such as cottonseed, soybean, corn and safflower. Sunflower and sesame seeds, walnuts and pecans are also high in polyunsaturates.

Polyunsaturate fats are usually soft or liquid at room temperature.

Monounsaturated fats, like olive oil, have been found to lower high blood pressure (*Journal of the American Medical Association* 257:3251-56). At Stanford Medical School, Dr. Stephen Fortmann has found that one tablespoon of olive oil per day equalled a 3.1 drop in systolic (the upper number) pressure. If three tablespoons of olive oil or other monounsaturated fats were added to the daily diet or substituted for saturated fats, the systolic pressure could drop up to 9.4 points and the diastolic pressure could be reduced by 6.3 points, Fortmann claims. So increasing your monounsaturated fats while decreasing your saturated fats should help lower your blood pressure naturally.

Blood pressure drops significantly when the amount of fat is reduced to less than 40 percent of the diet, according to research by Dr. James M. Iacono of the U.S. Department of Agriculture. Use these tips to help reduce your cholesterol level and lower your blood pressure.

> Do not consume more than 100 milligrams of cholesterol for each 1,000 calories. Daily cholesterol should not exceed 300 milligrams.

> Saturated fats, found in red meats and dairy products, should be reduced to less than 10 percent of total calories. Foods that are rich in cholesterol should be avoided or drastically limited in the diet. These foods include: egg yolks, organ meats and most cheeses. Foods that should be reduced because they are high in saturated fats include: butter, bacon, beef, whole milk, cream, chocolate, almost any food of animal origin, hydrogenated vegetable shortenings, coconut oil and palm oil.

> Unsaturated fats, such as fish and vegetable oils, may constitute as much as 10 percent of total calories.

> Total fat intake should be less than 30 percent of your daily calories.

> Try to avoid artificial and non-dairy creamers. If you need to use a powdered product (due to lack of refrigeration) use low-fat powdered milk. The instant, non-fat dry milk is convenient and has a lower fat content than a non-dairy cream substitute.

> Don't use foods containing coconut or palm oil. They are high in saturated fats.

> Cut back on beef, lamb and pork. Never eat any combination of them more than three times per week.

> Don't eat duck, goose or organ meats. They are high in fat content.

> If you must eat beef, use only lean cuts. When cooking at home, cut off all visible fat. Broiling, baking or roasting the meat in its own juices are the healthiest methods of preparation. When eating out, select the best quality cuts like a filet mignon or chateaubriand. Keep your portions small and don't use any gravy or sauce. Also, avoid casseroles and pot pies.

> When preparing chicken or turkey, be sure to cut off the skin because much of the fat is contained in the skin. Eat the light meat on a turkey or chicken because it contains less fat than the dark meat.

> When eating red meat, serve less meat by preparing dishes that use meat plus vegetables, pasta or grains. Then you can use less meat per person while still providing adequate protein, vitamins and minerals. Stir-frying strips of meat with vegetables or cooking them in a wok is a good example.

> For dishes that require hamburger, substitute ground turkey (without the skin) or, if you are a hunter, you may want to substitute ground venison.

> Don't buy meat, fish or poultry that is already breaded. If you want to bread the meat, make your

own breading with plain bread crumbs, herbs, skim milk and egg whites. Don't deep-fry after breading.

> Avoid prepared luncheon meats. As well as being high in fat, they are high in sodium and nitrites. Sliced turkey breast, tuna salad and salmon salad (without mayonnaise) are good luncheon alternatives.

> When making soup, chili, or stew, place the broth in the refrigerator overnight. In the morning, remove any fat that has hardened at the top.

> Eliminate bacon bits from your diet. In salads and soups, try homemade croutons or herbs to add that "spicy" taste.

> Limit your egg yolks to two per week. This includes not only whole eggs, but eggs used in baking and cooking. To reduce cholesterol, *Cardiac Alert* (9:5) recommends using two egg whites instead of one whole egg in cooking and baking.

> If you are using egg substitutes in trying to reduce your cholesterol intake, be careful. Many commercial egg substitutes are high in sodium or high in fat, even though they may be cholesterol-free.

The American Heart Association recommends making a cholesterol-free egg substitute especially for use in baking: Beat three egg whites. Then add one-fourth cup non-fat milk, one tablespoon non-fat dry milk powder, and one teaspoon of polyunsaturated vegetable oil. Mix these four ingredients together to make a healthful egg substitute. According to an avid cholesterol-watcher, if you add a drop of yellow food coloring when making French toast, your family won't be able to tell the difference!

> Pre-packaged cake mixes, biscuits and pancake mixes are usually made with eggs. To make your own easy mix, combine all the necessary dry ingredients together and freeze. When you want to bake them, just take your mix out of the freezer and add the liquids. For the liquids, use only egg substitutes, non-fat milk and vegetable oils.

> When buying pasta, avoid noodles made with eggs.

> Avoid crackers that contain lard or "animal fat". Study the list of ingredients and buy only crackers made with acceptable vegetable oils. If a cracker leaves a grease stain on a paper towel, it contains too much lard.

> Avoid croissants.

> When buying bagels, choose those made with water rather than eggs.

> Switch from butter to margarine, preferably

soft margarine. People usually use less soft margarine because it is easier to spread, so it is the best choice.

> Don't use saturated fat like lard, shortening, or animal fat drippings for cooking. Use polyunsaturated oil like corn, safflower, sesame seed, cottonseed, soybean and sunflower oils. Monounsaturated oil like olive oil is best for your health, according to recent studies. Polyunsaturated oils like corn, safflower, seasame seed, cottonseed, soybean and sunflower oils are better for your heart and arteries than saturated fat, but not quite as good as monounsaturated oils.

> Eliminate one pie crust when baking pies. Make your pies "open-faced" rather than covering them with a second crust.

> In recipes, reduce the amount of added fat by one-third to one-half. Make up the difference by adding water. For example, if a recipe calls for one cup of oil, just add two-thirds cup of oil and one-third cup water. The next time you make the same recipe, try further reducing the amount of oil. Keep cutting back on the fat until you have reached the "lowest possible" fat level for that recipe.

> For sautéing, use a vegetable spray. The spray

will limit the amount of fat you'll use in cooking.

> Avoid butter or sour cream on baked potatoes. Eating a plain baked potato is good for you and low in fat!

> Substitute low-fat cottage cheese or nonfat yogurt for sour cream in your favorite recipes.

> Avoid avocadoes and olives.

> Reduce the amount of peanut butter in your diet or eliminate it entirely.

> Eliminate potato chips, french fries and all fried "fast food" from your diet. When eating out, pull off all the crisp, breaded portions from fried foods because they become saturated with cooking oil.

> Eliminating salt and butter or oil on popcorn is not always easy because without the liquid, it seems as if no other herbs or spices will stick to the popcorn. Try this delicious alternative. Lightly spray the popcorn with a "non-stick" vegetable spray, then add cinnamon, curry powder, onion powder (not onion salt), chili powder or other herbs for an enjoyable flavor without cholesterol or salt.

> If you want cheese, eat moderate amounts of the low-fat varieties like Mozzarella, Provolone and Swiss.

For the taste of cheese, try a sprinkle of grated Parmesan cheese. It will still give you a cheese flavor but it contains fewer grams of fat.

> Avoid heavy salad dressings like blue cheese. Try to eat less salad dressing by placing the dressing on the side and using it only as necessary.

> Drink skim or low-fat milk. Avoid using whole milk, evaporated milk, or sweetened, condensed milk. If you want the convenience of condensed milk, use a low-fat evaporated milk powder.

> Switch from ice cream to ice milk, sherbet, sorbet or frozen fruit treats. Beware of frozen yogurt, unless it is frozen low-fat yogurt.

> Limit your intake of baking chocolate or milk chocolate which contains highly saturated cocoa butter. Substitute cocoa powder for chocolate when possible in recipes. The American Heart Association recommends substituting three tablespoons cocoa powder and one tablespoon polyunsaturated oil for each one ounce piece of baking chocolate. It will cut the amount of saturated fat by over sixty percent.

> Try scallops. They are a low-fat and low-cholesterol seafood. Avoid lobster and shrimp.

> Avoid all foods prepared with sauces or gravies like a cheese sauce (described as "au gratin"),

hollandaise sauce, lobster sauce, sweet and sour sauce, mayonnaise or regular gravy. Tomato sauce may also be high in salt!

> When buying processed foods, look for "catch words" on the label that indicate high fat or high cholesterol levels: lard, butter, shortening, fat, cream, hydrogenated or hardened oils, palm, palm kernel oil, coconut oil, whole-milk solids, whole-milk fat, egg solids, egg-yolk solids, suet, animal fat, animal byproducts, cocoa butter, milk chocolate, or imitation milk chocolate. Avoid these products.

> Check food labels very carefully. Products labeled "low-cholesterol" may not conform to the same standards and could be high in saturated fats.

> Eat chick-peas, soybean products, oats, and carrots to help maintain low cholesterol levels. Oat bran is an excellent source of water-soluble fiber and can reduce blood cholesterol levels by 6 to 19 percent, based on data from the Lipid Research Clinic. Researchers at Northwestern University (*Journal of the American Dietetic Association*) discovered that about two cups of oatmeal or two oat bran muffins daily, combined with moderate levels of dietary fat and cholesterol, can lower cholesterol levels in just a few weeks. If you prefer oat bran muffins, be sure to

use a low cholesterol substitute, rather than eggs, in the muffins.

For best overall health, also eat foods like fruit, bran, whole grain breads and cereals. These foods may not lower cholesterol as well as oat bran does, but they are better than oat bran for preventing colon cancer and other diseases.

Because diet is so important to your health and especially your blood pressure, we have prepared a 14-day diet plan (see Appendix Two) and a series of recipes for a low fat diet (Appendix Three).

The Role of Vitamins and Minerals

Protective Potassium

There is evidence that potassium may help protect against high blood pressure. Part of the evidence, however, is clouded by the fact that societies which have high levels of salt consumption also have low levels of potassium consumption and vice versa.

A recent study at Duke University showed a significant drop in blood pressure in just two months when participants were given potassium. Although potassium lowered blood pressure in most individuals, blood pressure dropped the most in blacks.

Potassium supplementation is extremely important in treating blood pressure problems in blacks, the doctors concluded in *Hypertension* (9:571-5).

Since this and other research indicates that supplemental potassium in the diet may help to lower blood pressure, it may be beneficial to eat more foods like bananas and citrus fruits, especially grapefruit, which are relatively high in potassium. Potassium is also widely distributed in foods like cantaloupe, potatoes, raisins, pineapple juice, tomatoes, pears, apple juice, peaches, apples, meat, milk and nuts.

People taking some diuretic drugs that reduce natural potassium will also receive a prescription for a potassium supplement. See potassium supplement in Chapter 8.

Adults need 1525-5625 mg. of potassium daily, according to the U.S. Recommended Dietary Allowance. Potassium supplements should not be used by people who have kidney disease or who are taking a prescription diuretic that is potassium-sparing, because excessive potassium can be harmful or even fatal. Large doses of potassium should be avoided unless prescribed by a doctor because high levels of potassium can cause heart attacks.

Additional Calcium

Calcium supplements may help to lower some cases of high blood pressure. According to new research published in *Drug Therapy* (16,11:63), many people do not get enough calcium. Inadequate calcium can lead to high blood pressure. Another study indicates that people with high blood pressure consume 20 to 25 percent less calcium than people who don't have high blood pressure. Signs of extremely low levels of calcium in the diet are muscle cramps and numbness in the limbs. Adequate vitamin D is necessary for the absorption of calcium.

Dr. Lawrence Resnick at the New York Hospital-Cornell Medical Center has found a link between people who are salt retentive and calcium supplementation. The more salt seems to affect someone's blood pressure, the more calcium supplements seem to improve their blood pressure, Resnick reports in the *Journal of Hypertension* (4:5182-5). Blacks and older people seem to benefit from calcium most, he says.

According to the *Journal of the American Medical Association* 257:1772-6), blood pressure dropped a "modest but significant" amount when men with normal blood pressure levels took 1,500 mg. of calcium daily, according to research by Purdue University professor, Roseann Lyle, Ph.D.

Another study, by researchers from Johns Hopkins University School of Medicine, confirmed that the "degree to which blood pressure falls depends on the amount of calcium taken." Although blood pressure usually rises in the last trimester of pregnancy, blood pressure levels remained constant in women who received 1,500 milligrams of calcium per day *(Obstetrics and Gynecology)*.

The risk of high blood pressure can be reduced by 22 percent in women who take 800 milligrams of calcium (the RDA) a day, reports a new study from Harvard Medical School. Blood pressure in women taking 800 milligrams per day was compared to women taking just 400 milligrams per day. Nutritionists have warned that most American women are not getting the RDA in their diets. They recommend either changing the diet by increasing low-fat dairy products, like skim milk, cottage cheese and yogurt, or taking daily calcium supplements.

Since taking calcium supplements or increasing the amount of calcium in the diet has few harmful side effects, extra calcium could be part of a blood pressure reducing therapy. Many people do not get the Recommended Daily Allowance set by the U.S. government. So the supplements should not be "megadoses" but enough to meet our daily requirements. To avoid overdosing on calcium, increase the amount of caclium in the diet rather than relying on supplements. The RDA of calcium is 800 — 1200 mg. per day for adult males and females. Dairy products, salmon, sardines and leafy green vegetables are the best natural sources of calcium.

Calcium supplementation should be avoided by people who have calcium oxalate kidney stones or by those with high blood-levels of calcium which make them more inclined to develop kidney stones.

Excessive amounts of calcium and vitamin D may make it difficult for the body to eliminate extra calcium, which can cause problems. Excessive vitamin D can be dangerous and actually can cause high blood pressure by promoting the formation of deposits in the arteries. The Recommended Dietary Allowance (RDA) of vitamin D is 400 IU (international units) per day. Anyone under medical care should consult with his physician before greatly increasing vitamin D or calcium supplementation.

Even if you start taking supplemental calcium, do not stop taking blood pressure medication except on your doctor's advice.

Supplementing Magnesium

A recent study by Dr. Burton M. Altura links low magnesium levels to high blood pressure. He believes that if the level of magnesium is too low, the calcium level becomes too high and the blood vessels contract, causing high blood pressure. In a separate study by Cornell University, Dr. Lawrence Resnick discovered that people with high blood pressure tend to have low magnesium in their red blood cells. Futhermore, Resnick claims that the patients who have their blood pressure under control have higher magnesium levels.

Another study in the *American Journal of Clinical Nutrition* (45:469-75) showed that older men who had the highest daily intake of magnesium had the lower blood pressure levels.

Other research shows that people have lower blood pressure if their water supplies have high concentrations of magnesium. Magnesium often is found with calcium in drinking water and in mineral supplements like Dolomite.

Whole-grain products, vegetables, black-eyed peas, bananas, apples, peaches, lima beans, seafood and peanuts are good sources of magnesium. The water supply is also an excellent source of magnesium in many areas of the country where the water is relatively hard. Adult males need between 350-400 mg. of magnesium daily, while adult women need about 300 mg. according to the recommended daily allowance set by the U.S. government.

Increasing Choline

Choline(a near vitamin) supplements are reported to help control blood pressure. In a clinical study, one-third of a group of patients with high blood pressure had their blood pressure return to normal after receiving choline supplements. When the supplements were discontinued, their blood pressure rose once again. However, additional studies are needed to confirm that choline alone was responsible.

Lecithin, soybeans, eggs, fish, liver and wheat germ are rich natural sources of choline. Green vegetables, peanuts, brewer's yeast, and sunflower seeds are also good sources.

Excess Vitamins

An overdose of vitamin D, from either excessive exposure to the sun, which acts on the skin to help produce vitamin D, or from taking high doses of vitamin D supplements, can lead to high blood pressure. Vitamin E, in doses larger than the RDA of twelve I.U.'s per day, can also cause high blood pressure.

Cadmium

Cadmium is a "heavy metal" which may be found in trace amounts in water supplies in the United States and in other countries. The cause and effect relationship between high levels of cadmium and high blood pressure exists as it does with salt. In studies at Dartmouth Medical School (*American Journal of Physiology* 214:469-74), Dr. Henry Schroeder found a direct link between cadmium and high blood pressure in rats. Cadmium is leeched into our water supply by soft water. Hard water does not seem to absorb cadmium as easily.

Your local water authority may be able to tell you if your water supply has higher than average concentrations of cadmium. If it does, using certified pure bottled water would be a good alternative.

Lead: Are you exposing your body to danger?

Lead poisoning can elevate blood pressure

(*Lancet* 2: 7975; 1-3 and *Medical Toxicology* 2:3; 210-232) and damage the brain, bones, kidneys, liver, central nervous system, and immune system, and cause slow learning in children. A recent study in *New England Journal of Medicine* (316:1037-43) found that children who were exposed to high lead levels before birth were physically and mentally impaired during their first two years of life.

Move away from plants that emit lead as industrial waste, or move to the country from the city. "*All* city residents" have slighter higher blood lead levels than people who live in the country, reports *Cardiac Alert* (Vol. 7 No. 7).

If you live in an older home and have soft water, have the lead level of your drinking water tested by the local EPA (Environmental Protection Agency). Soft water is slightly acidic and can leach lead from old pipes or fittings in and connected to your home. Evan T. Smith, a mechanical engineer from Idaho, suggests running tap water for a few minutes before using it because stagnant water has the highest lead content. By just flushing the pipes with fresh water, you will be able to use water with a lower lead content. If you know that your water pipes are soldered with lead, have them replaced.

The lead content in paint is now carefully regulated, but paint on the walls, molding and bannisters of old homes, could contain high levels of lead. Children and pregnant women should avoid remodeling of older homes where high levels of lead may be found. Do not burn painted boards in an indoor fireplace or woodstove, because the lead from the paint would be dispersed into the air.

People who repair car radiators have been lead-poisoned due to poor ventilation and a lack of safety procedures, reports the New England Journal of Medicine (317: 214-8). The doctors warn that anyone working in auto repairs should properly ventilate the work area and take breaks outdoors at least once each hour.

People who manufacture batteries, remodel old homes, or work in smelting are at increased risk of lead poisoning. Be sure to clean these work clothes thoroughly and separately from other clothes. Shower, scrub and change into clean clothes as soon as your work day is over.

Avoid indoor shooting ranges. The fine lead particles expelled in shooting can contribute to lead poisoning, the Journal of the American Medical Association (259:1385) reports. Frequent vacuuming of the firing range can help reduce the risk.

Many cases of lead poisoning are caused by frequent use of an everyday item, like a coffee mug that is cracked or improperly glazed and allows lead to leach into your beverage, especially if you drink acidic beverages. Do not store highly acidic foods or beverages in ceramic ware. The acid in the food or drink reacts with the glaze and increases the lead content of the food. The Merck Manual especially warns about the storage of wine, cider, fruits, fruit juices, tomatoes, tomato juice, and cola drinks because they are highly acidic.

Do not use pottery or leaded glass from local craftspeople to serve or store food. Beware of imported pottery. The Food and Drug Administration (FDA) has regulated the lead content in serving ware, pewter, enamelware and pottery since the early 1970s. However, many ceramic products that are imported into the U.S., souvenir plates, or products made by local craftspeople may not meet safety standards. Plates with high lead content can be used "for decorative purposes only" but should not come in contact with food.

Do not drink homemade wine or whiskey. Homemade liquor often has a high lead content because facilities and ingredients are not inspected and may not follow lead content standards.

Use only lead-free gasoline in your vehicles, even if you have an older car or truck. If you use leaded gas, you are contributing to the lead pollution problem.

A Note About Vitamin C

People trying to reduce their salt intake should avoid taking sodium ascorbate. Sodium ascorbate is a formulation of vitamin C that contains sodium. If you need a vitamin C supplement while cutting back on sodium, ascorbic acid or calcium ascorbate forms of vitamin C are preferred.

The Effect of Alcohol

Excessive alcohol drinking is the leading cause of high blood pressure among men who drink more than one ounce of alcohol (two drinks) per day. Alcohol makes blood pressure skyrocket as it damages the liver and kidneys and causes fluid build-up, says Dr. Arthur Klastsy at Kaiser Permanente Medical Center in Oakland, CA. Klastsy found that one or two drinks a day didn't affect the blood pressure, but excessive drinking caused blood pressure to rise dramatically

(*Annals of Internal Medicine* 98:846-848).

Researchers at Harvard Medical School recently confirmed that blood pressure in women was also affected by heavy drinking. If 30 to 34 grams of alcohol, the equivalent of two mixed drinks or three glasses of wine, was consumed daily, women increased their risk of developing high blood pressure by 40 percent. The risk jumped to 90 percent in women who drank more than 34 grams of alcohol each day, reports researcher Charles Hennekens, M.D.

Another study found that older men and women were more likely to have their blood pressure increased by heavy drinking (*American Journal of Epidemiology* 118:497-507). The researchers were not sure if the increase was caused by a different reaction to alcohol in older people or if alcohol has a cumulative effect after many years of heavy drinking.

Drinking just two alcoholic drinks per day can undo all the blood-pressure reducing effects of exercising, a new study at the Medical College of Wisconsin revealed. So don't exercise and then drink alcoholic beverages.

Since heavy drinking is also known to increase

heart problems, the American Heart Association is urging people not to drink more than two drinks per day to lower their high blood pressure and protect their heart. High blood pressure that is caused solely by high alcohol consumption usually disappears within a few weeks of giving up alcohol.

Taking Garlic

In studies at the University of Vienna, Dr. F.G. Piotrousky discovered that garlic reduced blood pressure in about forty percent of his high blood pressure patients, reports *The Vitamin Bible*.

Other work at Loma Linda University in California has shown that four grams of garlic a day helped reduced blood fats in people with high cholesterol levels.

Researchers are not sure exactly why garlic lowers blood pressure and cholesterol. Eric Block, Ph.D., of the State University of New York at Albany, says the key to garlic's benefits is in its most active anti-clotting ingredient called ajoene.

Since garlic can cause bad breath and body odor, *The Vitamin Bible* recommends taking it in perles which release in your intestines rather than your stomach. Researchers in Japan have produced another alternative called kyolic. *Prevention* magazine reports that kyolic provides the beneficial elements of garlic, is "odor-modified" and lowers blood fats without the odoriferous side effects.

Caffeine

Caffeine can raise blood pressure significantly and should be avoided. Caffeine consumption may create a false number of high blood pressure patients because caffeine raises borderline blood pressure levels, David Robertson, M.D. reported in the *New England Journal of Medicine* (298:181-186). Other studies in the *American Journal of Cardiology* (53:918-22) have found that systolic and diastolic blood pressure levels were raised an average of nine points with just two cups of coffee.

Caffeine is found in most "cola" and "pepper" drinks, some diet pills, coffee, tea and chocolate.

Black Licorice

Black licorice or licorice extracts should be avoided if you suffer from high blood pressure, according to researchers at Tufts University. Black licorice can make the body hold on to salt, lose potassium and cause fluid retention *(New England Journal of Medicine* (278:1381-3). People taking diuretics for their high blood pressure should be especially careful to avoid licorice because it seems to compound the problems and bad side effects of diuretic drugs. About 90 percent of the licorice imported into the United States is used in chewing tobacco. This is another reason people with high blood pressure should avoid all forms of tobacco.

Conclusion

The foods we eat and drink are such a major factor in causing high blood pressure that they can help us gain control over the disease rather than letting it control us. It takes knowledge and willpower to change our eating habits, but the payoff is far greater than any effort it takes to change. Not only will you feel better physcially, but you will have the satisfaction that you have won the upper hand in your battle against high blood pressure if you take control of your diet.

Chapter Six

Lifestyle Factors in Lowering Blood Pressure

In the last chapter you learned that what you put into your body — what you eat and drink— greatly affects your blood pressure. In this chapter you will look at how you treat your body — your lifestyle — and how that affects your blood pressure.

Obesity: How much weight are you making your body carry?

Blood pressure levels increase in proportion to the number of pounds someone is overweight, according to researchers who studied the residents of Framingham, Massachusetts, for more than ten years. It is more difficult for the heart to pump the blood in an overweight person because the heart must pump more blood through more tissue.

But how heavy is too heavy? Most medical professionals describe obesity as being twenty to forty percent heavier than your ideal weight. However, health professionals warn that if you are ten pounds over your ideal weight, you are overweight. About one-fourth of the U.S. population is more than twenty percent over desired weight, according to the Centers for Disease Control in Atlanta.

Since the heavier you are, the higher your risk of developing high blood pressure, obesity is one of the major causes of high blood pressure. However, the Framingham study also found that blood pressure dropped significantly when weight was lost. So just by gaining or losing weight, you can affect your blood pressure.

Remember that measuring pounds and ounces is not the only way to determine who is fat. Body builders, athletes and people who do hard manual labor are often heavier than their "ideal" weight, but they are not overweight. Since muscle weighs more than fat, you can be heavier without being fat. If you can "pinch an inch" you need to lose weight. The pinch test can be used on the underneath of your upper arm or on your stomach. However, usually the pinch test is not necessary because most people know when they are overweight. The hard part is just admitting it to ourselves and doing something about it.

People with mild high blood pressure who lost just ten pounds were able to stop taking medicine to control their blood pressure in a recent study, according to *Better Health* (Vol.5 No.8). A different research team found a direct relationship with the amount of weight lost and the reduction in blood pressure. They found that with every seven pounds lost, the top number (systolic blood pressure level) will drop seven points and the bottom number (diastolic) will drop four points.

What is your ideal weight?

It is determined by your age, height and sex. The weight chart that follows is based on the life-expectancy by sex at certain ages, weights and heights. They show that "ideal" weights increase as we get older.

Weight Table For Men and Women, Based on Age and Height*

Height Feet and Inches	Acceptable Weight Range (in pounds) 35Yr	45 Yr	55 Yr	65 Yr
4 10	92-119	99-127	107-135	115-142
4 11	95-123	103-131	111-139	119-147
5 0	98-127	106-135	114-143	123-152
5 1	101-131	110-140	118-148	127-157
5 2	105-136	113-144	122-153	131-163
5 3	108-140	117-149	126-158	135-168
5 4	112-145	121-154	130-163	140-173
5 5	115-149	125-159	134-168	144-179
5 6	119-154	129-164	138-174	148-184
5 7	122-159	133-169	143-179	153-190
5 8	126-163	137-174	147-184	158-196
5 9	130-168	141-179	151-190	162-201
5 10	134-173	145-184	156-195	167-207
5 11	137-178	149-190	160-201	172-213
6 0	141-183	153-195	165-207	177-219
6 1	145-188	157-200	169-213	182-225
6 2	149-194	162-206	174-219	187-232
6 3	153-199	166-212	179-225	192-238
6 4	157-205	171-218	184-231	197-244

*Table values are for height without shoes and weight without clothes.

Source: Baltimore Longitudinal Study of Aging, conducted at the Gerontology Research Center, National Institute on Aging.

How can you lose weight?

Eat fewer calories and exercise. Most obesity is caused by underexercise rather than overeating, according to a recent report by the U.S. Department of Health and Human Services. The combination of exercise with a proper diet is important to fight obesity. These are very simple rules that can contribute to safe, gradual weight-loss. However, most Americans seem to want a "pill" that they can take so they will be thinner in the morning. Losing weight is lifelong commitment to proper nutrition and regular exercise. It is not too difficult, although it may be a drastic change from a sedentary lifestyle.

Consult your doctor before starting any weight loss program, especially if you are pregnant, over 60 years old and need to lose 20 pounds or more, or have an immediate family member who has had a heart attack or diabetes.

Here are some tips on how to change your eating habits so you can lose weight and keep it off:

> Avoid crash diets and dangerous weight-loss schemes. Choose a diet that you can live with for the rest of your life. Once someone goes off a severe diet, they usually binge to meet all their cravings that have not been fulfilled. Cycles of rapid weight loss,

weight gain, weight loss and weight gain are extremely hard on the body's organs, can lead to high blood pressure and can be dangerous to your overall health. Gradual weight loss that can be maintained is the healthiest way to lose weight.

> Keep a food journal of what, how much and when you eat each day. With a journal you can see exactly where your calories and nutrition are coming from and how you can alter your eating habits.

> Weigh yourself once a week and record it in your food journal. Daily fluctuations in weight are not reliable, but a weekly weighing will allow you to evaluate if your program is working.

> Set a realistic goal weight for yourself, preferably with your doctor's endorsement. Being overweight is dangerous, but so is being underweight. Each person has a different metabolism that burns calories at slightly different rates. Choose a weight that is safe and healthy for your height, age and lifestyle.

> Choose specific times to eat your meals and snacks, and do not eat at any other time. Never skip meals because you will be inclined to eat more at the next meal to make up the difference.

> Do not eat if you are not hungry. As children,

we were often required to eat "everything on our plates" and ate even when we were not hungry, but these patterns can lead to obesity.

> Learn to say "no" without feeling guilty. Once again, do not let someone coerce you into eating.

> Eat slowly. Put your utensils down after each bite. It takes several minutes for the stomach to tell the brain that it is full, so eating slowly will help you to realize you're full before you overeat.

> Try to reduce your intake of all food rather than completely restricting yourself to certain foods. If you are not allowed to have a specific item, usually you will crave that "forbidden fruit." This is particularly true when working with overweight children. It is best to learn good overall eating habits rather than prohibiting certain foods for the rest of their lives.

> Drink grapefruit juice, unsalted (a low sodium brand) tomato juice or unsweetened lemonade as an appetizer before your meal. If you allow 20 minutes before you eat, the acid in the juice will help you feel full, and you will be able to eat less. Drink the juice of a whole lemon squeezed into a glass of water, twice a day, for another natural appetite suppressant.

> Serve your meals on smaller plates so they will look fuller.

> Place the food on the plates away from the table. If you bring serving dishes to the table, you will be more tempted to have additional helpings.

> Avoid dishes and table settings that are bright because bright colors may stimulate the appetite.

> Never eat food out of the original container. Take out an appropriate serving and return the container to its proper place. By eating directly out of the container, you are more likely to eat too much.

> Try to leave something on your plate. In some oriental countries this is considered a high compliment because it shows that you have had plenty to eat. If you have been raised to clear your plate and not to "waste food," learning to leave a small portion on your plate will be good for you.

> Switch to lower calorie foods like skim milk and calorie-reduced products.

> Many doctors now recommend avoiding products with artificial sweeteners. Although they seem to be a boon for dieters, some doctors believe that artificial sweeteners increase or maintain the desire for sweets which is not helpful to someone who is dieting.

Using artificial sweeteners does not guarantee weight loss, reports new research by the American

Cancer Society. In a study of 78,000 dieters, people using artificial sweeteners gained more weight than people not using substitutes. The artificial sweeteners did not cause the weight gain. However, the researchers concluded that the people thought they were cutting back by using the artificial sweeteners, and they just didn't limit their calories overall. Don't be lulled into a false sense of security — reducing total caloric intake and exercising are the only true ways to lose weight.

> Avoid diet pills, even prescription drugs, unless your doctor believes they are absolutely necessary. Recently a 37-year old woman nearly died when her heart stopped, Dr. Harry R. Gibbs reports in the *New England Journal of Medicine* (318: 17, 1127). The woman had been taking three drugs prescribed for weight loss — phentermine hydrochloride, thyroid, and trichlormethiazide — and didn't have any heart or artery problems. Gibbs warns that using inappropriate prescription drugs to treat obesity, even in someone without heart problems, can lead to "sudden catastrophic events."

> Do not use over-the-counter appetite suppressants. One common ingredient, phenylpropanolamine hydrochloride (PPA) has been found to cause high

blood pressure even at the doses recommended for weight loss. Anyone with diabetes, heart disease, thyroid disease or high blood pressure should avoid products containing PPA, recommends the *Health Letter* (2:1).

> Do not use or purchase a product that promises to reduce or remove fat in one specific body area. Except for specific exercise or cosmetic surgery, one part of your body cannot be reduced.

> Do not use a "body wrap" in hopes of losing weight. The only weight loss that body wraps provide is the loss of sweat which is just temporary. Using body wraps can be harmful because the body's temperature is allowed to escalate.

> Eat more vegetables and smaller portions of meat, especially if it's red meat.

> Trim all noticeable fat from meat, and remove the skin before eating.

> Eat plenty of high-fiber foods like whole-grain products, beans and vegetables.

> Use a low calorie, soft-spread alternate to butter. If you use a soft-spread, you'll use less because it spreads easier than butter or margarine.

> Eliminate alcohol because it is high in "empty" calories. Alcohol products contain a lot of calories,

but they have no nutritional value. Alcohol consumption is also a contributing factor in high blood pressure.

> Keep healthful snacks available. Try cutting up celery, carrots, broccoli, cauliflower, radishes and whatever other vegetables you like and leaving them in the refrigerator. Buy plenty of fruit. It provides quick and easy snacks.

> Buy high-quality popcorn that tastes good without butter or salt. To flavor your popcorn, try lightly spraying the popcorn with a low calorie vegetable oil, then add cinnamon, curry powder, onion powder, chili powder or other herbs.

> Reduce or eliminate high calorie nuts and nut products, including peanut butter.

> Never go grocery shopping when you are hungry. If you are hungry, you will tend to buy more, and you are more easily tempted to buy high-calorie foods.

> Make a shopping list of things you need and stick to it. Don't be seduced by unnecessary foods.

> Don't keep high-calorie foods in your home.

> Don't store food within sight.

> Eat early in the day to achieve your maximum weight loss. Researchers at Tulane Unversity found

that people who ate their last meal at least eight hours before they went to sleep lost between five and ten pounds a month (*Postgraduate Medicine* 79:4,352). The participants did not change the amount of food they ate, or the number of calories, just the time of day it was eaten. If you eat most of your daily calories in the morning and at noon, and have a light snack for the evening meal, you should be able to boost your weight loss.

> The Good Wellness Program for Weight Management suggests placing a bottle of mouthwash in front of the refrigerator door. If you stray into the kitchen looking for "something to eat," you will have to move the mouthwash first. The director of the program, suggests rinsing with the mouthwash to satisfy the cravings without consuming any calories.

> Brushing your teeth frequently may help reduce snacking. Your teeth and mouth feel so good that you don't have the desire to eat.

> Remember your diet when eating outside of your home, at a restaurant, or someone else's home. If you eat at a cafeteria, like a school lunchroom, check with the food services manager to see if low-calorie meals can be ordered.

> If you must have dessert, try sharing it with one

or two other people. After a fine meal, you do not need the dessert, but a small sample may meet your craving for a sweet.

> When flying or traveling by train, request a low-calorie meal at least 24 hours in advance of your departure.

> Do not reward yourself with food or use food to fight stress or depression. Buy yourself a gift or treat yourself to a favorite activity, rather than using food as a release or reward.

> Try squeezing your earlobe for sixty seconds before eating. This is a technique of acupressure that may help curb your appetite.

> Obese dieters who lose weight very quickly are at increased risk of developing gallstones, doctors at the Cedars-Sinai Medical Center in Los Angeles report. However, if four aspirin are taken each day, the dieter should not develop gallstones, according to the research. You should discuss the aspirin treatment with your doctor if you are considering a low-calorie diet.

> Exercise alone does not cause weight to "just disappear." However, a regular exercise program will make it easier for you to maintain your weight. Since the most important element of exercising is

actually "doing it," it is important that the exercise you choose is something you will continue. According to the Federal Trade Commission, of the people who join a fitness club or health spa, 70 percent will quit within just three months.

Exercise helps some people lose weight because it increases their awareness of their bodies. Many people who start an exercise program are suddenly aware of what and how much they are eating. Exercising (and feeling those tired muscles) can be a good reminder that they are trying to lose weight. If you are faithful to your exercise program, you'll eat better and eat less because you won't want to "undo" the good your exercising has done!

For more practical help in losing weight and lowering blood pressure, we've compiled a menu plan for two weeks and recipes for healthy foods. Please refer to Appendices Two and Three in the back of the book.

Stress: How much emotional strain do you put on your body?

Anxiety, frustration and anger may aggravate "reactive" high blood pressure. With "reactive" high blood pressure, the body reacts to stressful situations by pumping adrenalin and speeding up the heart, sending more blood to the brain and muscles. The blood pressure rises and the liver dumps cholesterol into the bloodstream.

Being unhappy at work can raise your blood pressure, researchers at the University of Pittsburgh discovered. In a study of 288 men who had blue collar jobs, the researchers found that the more dissatisfied the worker was with his job, the higher his risk of having high blood pressure. If the man felt insecure about his job, had little opportunity for promotion, didn't feel part of the decision-making process or that the other employees were not supportive, he was more likely to have high blood pressure. Job stress and job dissatisfaction has also been linked to an increased risk of heart and artery diseases, reports the *American Journal of Epidemiology*.

However, many calm people have high blood pressure. Although it is a cause in some cases, you do not have to be under a lot of stress or be a "tense" person to have high blood pressure.

Learn to recognize your body's stress signals. Do you start to snap or lose your temper with loved ones? Are you more tired? Do unimportant little things start to bother you? Do you get headaches or body aches? Do you suffer from insomnia? Many of these symptoms plus clenched fists, chain smoking, biting your lips, sleeping too much, being quick to cry, and wanting to run away are all common signs of too much personal stress. The first step to alleviating stress is to learn to recognize its signs. Recognizing that you are under stress and seeking to help reduce the stress are very important.

How can you reduce stress? It's impossible to completely eliminate emotional strain, but it is possible to avoid some stressful situations. Talking it out, working off your anger, taking time out for yourself, doing for others and learning to tackle one job at at time are only a few of the positive actions you can take to lower your emotional tension.

Certain events, both good and bad, are known to be stressful. Researchers Holms and Rahe have rated several life events, starting with the most stressful. Some of these events are planned and some are sudden and cannot be anticipated. The top ten life events that cause stress, according to Holms and Rahe, are:

1. Death of a spouse.
2. Divorce.

3. Marital separation.
4. Jail term.
5. Death of a close family member.
6. Personal injury or illness.
7. Marriage.
8. Getting fired from work.
9. Marital reconciliation.
10. Retirement.

Whenever possible, try not to plan too many high-stress items at the same time. For example, getting married causes stress. If you buy a home, get married and start a new job all at the same time, you will be under a great deal of stress. However, if you can plan the events so they don't happen together, you can reduce your stress level.

Techniques for stress management should be appropriate for the kind of stress you experience. Physical methods like deep breathing and exercise should be used to cope with physical reactions to stress, like body aches, hyperactivity and the jitters. Mental calming methods should be used for mental stress.

Accept your own personal limitations. Accept the limitations of money; you will always want more than you have, and you may have to sacrifice some things to get what is important to you. Accept the limitations of your situation. If your plane is delayed or if you are stuck in a traffic jam, worrying and getting angry will not make the situation disappear.

Your approach to life has a lot to do with how much stress you create for yourself. For example, if you are a perfectionist about your own work and expect others to adhere to your high standards, you are setting yourself up for plenty of stress-filled days. Learning to accept things that are "less than perfect" could be important for your health. You don't have to completely leave your standards. Even if you accept a few "less than perfect" projects, you will lower your stress. Also, remember your strengths and weaknesses. No one can do all things well. Try to improve your strengths and your weaknesses. Don't be too hard on yourself when you discover that you cannot excel at everything.

Cool your competitive edge. Rather than constantly comparing yourself to others, set your own goals based on your own performance. Don't be constantly trying to get the best parking space, or get ahead of "that" car in traffic. Many times these minor competitions contribute to unnecessary stress in our lives.

Acknowledge your successes. Celebrate the things you accomplish, no matter how small. If you have a job that is repetitious, and it is difficult to see any progress, create and celebrate your own accomplishments.

If you always seem to be concerned with yourself, try reaching out to others. Doing something for someone else may help to put your problems into better perspective. Hopefully, you will become less self-centered as you appreciate the people around you.

Take time for yourself everyday. Do something that you enjoy.

Don't try to bear other people's stress. Women in traditional roles are famous for this. The wife and mother often tries to carry the burdens of her husband and children, and she feels very stressed. Learn to recognize that their problems are not your fault. You can be supportive and loving without carrying their stress.

Don't be afraid to get help. Asking for help is not a sign of weakness, but rather a sign that you know your own limitations. Many people are afraid to ask for help, and then the stress of the burdens they are carrying becomes overwhelming.

Don't be afraid to cry. Research has shown that crying is a natural and healthy way to deal with stress. Crying helps focus your emotions and provides a needed release. For crying to be most helpful, though, it must be done in private. You should be comfortable and be able to cry as long as you'd like.

Music is now being recognized, and used by professional therapists, to help relieve and treat stress. According to Alicia Gibbons, Ph.D., the past president of the National Association for Music Therapy, music can change the breathing rate, the heart rate and the level of stress someone is experiencing. Dr. Gibbons suggests that whatever music you prefer, the music that causes you to relax will be most helpful.

Songs from your past, that you associate with good times, can bring back those good feelings. However, the therapist prefers music without lyrics so you don't get caught up in listening to the words. After having a stressful experience, just lying down with your eyes closed and listening to the music should alleviate some of the symptoms of stress. The Sharper Image® and other companies sell tapes of "relaxing sounds" like gentle waves breaking on a shore.

Music can also help prepare a person for a

stressful situation. For example, if someone dreads going to a dentist or has an important business meeting, they can play their "calming" music on the way there. The right music can help you approach stressful events in a calm and serene manner.

If you have a stressful job, try to avoid bringing that stress home to your family. Taking your frustrations out on your family and friends may add to their stress, says Dr. Barbara Mackoff. There is a place for discussing your problems with your family, and your family should be able to support you. But learn the difference between having their support and making them share the burden of your stress.

Talk. Share your concerns, your fears, your dreams and your anxieties to your closest friend or spouse. Talking helps put the problems into correct perspective.

Some doctors, including Robert T. Johnson, M.D., author of *Stay Well*, recommend chamomile tea and tryptophan as natural relaxants. Others suggest taking CoA (pantothenate) for a natural relaxant.

Supplementation with vitamin C and iron, which is necessary for the formation of red blood cells which help carry oxygen to the body, may help fight stress. Stress may increase the need for niacin (vitamin B3) and thiamine (vitamin B1).

The best way to prepare your body to cope with stress is to get plenty of rest (seven to eight hours of sleep each night), avoid eating foods high in fats or salt, and eat nutritious foods. Researchers in France, and Dr. Burton M. Altura of Brooklyn, N.Y., have discovered that low magnesium levels make it more difficult to deal with stress, so be sure to get between 300 and 400 milligrams of magnesium daily. Avoid cigarettes, alcohol, caffeine and any other substances that are harmful to the body.

Chemists are now claiming that certain fragrances can help calm us in times of stress. Many cosmetic companies are marketing fragrance vials that contain "spiced apple" or other smells that are supposed to help us relax. In the South, pots of water containing special herbs and spices are kept on wood stoves, electric or gas ranges or over special candles to create a distinctive mood in the house. Research has proven that animals are greatly influenced by smells and aromas, but whether or not human beings can become relaxed just by breathing a certain scent is not known. However, if you have a certain aroma that you associate with peacefulness and calm, like the smell of hot apple pie baking in the oven, maybe fragrance therapy will help you relax.

Exercise, on your way home after work or as soon as you get home, can give you a chance to clear your mind as well as rejuvenate your body. Regular exercise will help improve your circulation, lower your blood pressure, and allow you to better cope with the stresses you face.

Develop your faith. If you believe in a benevolent God who is in control of the universe, concentrate on that fact. Remember that ultimately God is in charge of events, not you. Release your problems and turmoils to Him and look to Him for strength each day.

Exercise: What are you doing to strengthen your heart?

Blood pressure varies with the condition of the heart. Exercise which increases the strength of the heart may help to prevent or lower high blood pressure. Even mild exercise like walking can lower blood pressure *on the first day*, Dr. James M. Rippe, of the University of Massachusetts Medical School reports. In addition, exercise can also fight obesity, help you cope with stress, increase your self-esteem and reduce depression.

Since the heart is a muscle, it must be exercised like any other muscle to become stronger. If it is exercised regularly, its strength increases; if not, it becomes weaker. Although it is often believed that strenuous work harms the heart, scientific research has found no evidence that regular progressive exercise is harmful for the normal heart.

A strong heart muscle can pump a greater amount of blood with fewer strokes per minute. For example, the average individual has a resting heart rate of between seventy and eighty beats per minute, while a trained athlete may have a resting heart rate in the low fifties or even in the forties.

Before starting an exercise program consult a physician and follow a recommended plan. Remember to slowly increase the intensity and duration of exercise. Don't overdo it in the beginning. Watch for body signals, such as sharp pains and cramps, that tell you when you're doing too much.

Regular aerobic exercise, at least thirty consecutive minutes three times a week, is the key to better fitness. Aerobic exercise increases your endurance, helps improve circulation and strengthens the heart. Spurts of activity can actually be harmful to a nonactive person, so regularity and warm ups are important. Swimming, tennis, bicycling, rowing, skiing, jumping rope, aerobic dancing and hiking are some of the many aerobic activities that you can choose.

Walking is the number one form of exercise, and it is usually recommended by doctors as the best beginning exercise for people who are out of shape. Running is excellent for those who are in shape, but simple walking can help lower high blood pressure and improve your fitness level. If walking does not challenge you anymore, but you would like to continue, carry handweights. Small handweights, no more than five pounds per hand, will add to the upper body workout when walking and make your walk more beneficial.

The *Journal of the American Medical Association* (212;2267) says that people with high blood pressure should avoid isometrics. Isometrics are exercises that involve muscle contractions while the joints remain in place, like squeezing the hand against a fixed object. In the Journal, Dr. William S. Breall warns that isometrics can cause a temporary rise in blood pressure which can be extremely dangerous for people with blood pressure that is already high.

Sports physicians are now recommending

exercise that includes use of both the legs and the arms according to *Physician and Sports Medicine* (14:5,181). Window washers, farmers and orchestra conductors, all people who use their arms quite a bit daily, seem to have an increased life expectancy. For a complete workout that includes the arms, try swimming, cross-country skiing or using a rowing machine.

If you don't enjoy the type of exercise you are doing, you are less likely to make it a regular part of your daily life. *Consumer Guide®* has listed some principles that will help you choose a form of exercise that you will enjoy and continue to participate in. Before you start an exercise program, check with your doctor.

> Time. You must choose an activity that you are willing to devote time to every day or every other day. Downhill skiing may be something you enjoy, but if you can participate for only one day a week during three months of the year, you will need another form of exercise as well.

> Pleasure. The exercise you choose must be something you enjoy doing. Be willing to try several different activities at first so you don't limit yourself to what you have tried before. You may discover that

a form of exercise you thought would be boring is perfectly suited to your needs and enjoyment.

> Variety. Don't be afraid to choose a variety of activities that you enjoy. You may discover that aerobic classes during the week and a long walk or hike on the weekend mean a perfect combination for you.

> Success. Don't undermine your exercise by feeling guilty if you miss your planned activity. Look forward to your next time of exercise. Celebrate the successes you have enjoyed during your exercising. If you get discouraged, try doing the same routine or amount of exercise as your first time. You will find that it seems easy compared to what you can do after a period of regular exercise.

> Spouse. If you are married, having the support of your spouse can be very important. Finding an activity that you can do together can be great. However, if you can only find a form of exercise that your spouse will give you support in, that too can be important. Your spouse's support may make it easier for you to continue with regular exercise.

> Groups. Many people find that the support of a group makes regular exercise easier to continue. This doesn't mean you have to join an expensive

fitness club or take a class. Just getting a small group of friends who are willing to meet and go for a walk on a regular basis can help. The companionship of the group, knowing you are not alone, and enjoying exercise as a social activity are very helpful.

> Money. Some people find that a paid class is the best incentive for them to continue exercising. Even if you just have a little "miser" in you, you may feel the urge to attend all the classes because you don't want to "waste the money." If this works for you, keep paying for classes in advance!

Smoking: Are you habitually damaging your heart?

Smoking is a well-known hazard to people with high blood pressure. Smoking cigarettes, pipes or cigars can constrict the arteries, which directly raises high blood pressure and increases the risk of heart failure.

Chewing tobacco and snuff, also known as smokeless tobacco, should also be avoided because of their high salt content. According to an article in the *New England Journal of Medicine* (312: 919) the sodium levels in chewing tobacco and snuff are similar to the high levels found in dill pickles, which should also be avoided. Studies at Ohio State University have shown higher blood pressure levels in people who used smokeless tobacco, compared to nonusers. Smokeless tobacco also contains high amounts of licorice, another villain in the fight against high blood pressure. So you should avoid all forms of tobacco.

Many smokers continue smoking even when they realize it is bad for their health because nicotine is one of the most addictive substances used by human beings. It is extremely difficult for a smoker to quit smoking because of the physical craving for nicotine which is found with tobacco products.

Smoking is a learned behavior. Human beings do not have a "need" for the nicotine. The pressures of our peer groups and society have taught us to smoke. To quit smoking, you must "unlearn" this behavior and break the nicotine addiction.

The American Cancer Society, the American Lung Association, Merrell Dow Pharmaceuticals, Seventh Day Adventists and many other organizations have compiled these guidelines to help you "kick the habit":

> The *desire* to stop smoking will be your

biggest asset when you try to quit. If you don't want to quit, guidelines will not help.

> Examine your reasons for wanting to quit. Besides the physical damage of smoking, you may be helping your family and friends plus saving time and money. Write down at least ten reasons for quitting. Review these reasons daily and keep adding to the list.

> Decide you want to quit. Be positive about your decision. Then choose a quitting day and stick to it. If you are a heavy smoker while at work, you may want to quit on a Friday afternoon. By Monday morning, you'll have two smoke-less days behind you and should be better prepared for the stress of your first smoke-less work day.

> Identify the times and feelings you associate with smoking. You may smoke after meals, while you are under stress, or after sex. When possible, avoid the situations that you associate with smoking. If you feel the desire to smoke every time you have a cup of coffee or an alcoholic drink, cut out the coffee and alcohol as well. You may have to limit your social life until you feel secure about not smoking. Learning when you smoke and re-learning those activities without smoking, can be the most difficult

time in “kicking the habit.”

> Organize pleasant and busy activities for the day you will quit. Plan to do things with other people, preferably non-smokers. Keeping an active schedule may help you get over the first few days. You may want to have some kind of treat or celebration to start your non-smoking campaign.

> If you are quitting “cold turkey,” try to remove all temptations before you start. Throw away all cigarettes. Remove your ashtrays, lighters and matches. Don’t forget the ones you keep at work or in your purse.

> Keep your mouth clean. Brush and floss your teeth often so your mouth will taste clean and you won’t have as much urge to smoke. You may want to visit a dental hygienist and have your teeth cleaned within the first few days after you stop smoking. If you schedule the appointment beforehand, this appointment could be your first goal as a non-smoker.

> Some people find that sugar-free chewing gums also helps keep the mouth occupied if you have the urge to pick up a cigarette.

> If you miss having something in your hand to play with, try substituting a pen, pencil, or paper clip.

> If you feel the urge to smoke, do something

physical or take a bath or shower. Try doing more things with your hands, like writing letters, crafts, sewing, woodwork, housework or yardwork.

> Maintain or improve your physical health. Start regular exercise. Eat healthy meals, including lots of fruit and vegetables. Drink more fluids, including fruit juices and water. Everyone should drink at least eight glasses of water each day. Get lots of rest and relaxation. By getting your body in good condition, you will be more able to tolerate the physical symptoms of withdrawal from nicotine. Physical exercise will improve your breathing and blood flow, as well as provide a smoke-free activity.

> Get support. If your spouse smokes, try quitting together. You will be able to support and encourage each other. If not, try a local ex-smokers' group in your community. Learning about the hard times other people have experienced may make your troubles seem smaller. Involve someone else who will support you and you will improve the chances of becoming and staying a non-smoker.

> Remember that smoking is not just a bad habit. Smoking is also an addiction to the drug, nicotine. You may experience withdrawal symptoms. According to the U.S. Department of Health and Human

Services, mood changes, irritability, aggressiveness, anxiety, difficulty in sleeping, drowsiness, weight gain, lower blood pressure, headaches, upset stomachs and a decrease in the heart rate are common physical reactions to nicotine withdrawal. Usually, the withdrawal symptoms subside within a few days or a few weeks. Since they will end, don't let them stop you from achieving a smoke-free life!

Withdrawal from nicotine can be eased by a prescription drug chewing gum called Nicorette® which slowly releases a measured dose of nicotine into the system to reduce physical craving for tobacco products. Withdrawal from nicotine may also be eased by taking half a teaspoon of bicarbonate of soda in a glass of water two or three times a day. Apparently, the bicarbonate of soda helps hold nicotine in the system and reduces withdrawal symptoms by giving the body more time to adapt to withdrawal.

> While trying to stop smoking, Earl Mindell, author of *The Vitamin Bible,* recommends a variety of supplements to help overcome the withdrawal from nicotine. One tryptophan tablet, three times daily, seems to help reduce the irritability associated with nicotine withdrawal, he suggests. A good mulitvitamin, 100 mg. of a vitamin B complex, 100 mg. of

cysteine and 300 mg. of vitamin C will help keep the body healthy during the time you are withdrawing from nicotine, says Mindell.

> Don't try to have "just one" cigarette, for "old times" sake. Just like a "reformed" alcoholic, one cigarette can begin the smoking cycle again. Even in times of personal crisis, like the death of a loved one or the loss of a job, don't succumb to smoking.

> If you don't quit the first time you try, don't give up. Don't be too hard on yourself. There is a definite physical addiction to nicotine, and it may not be easy to stop. Some people need to try two or three times before they are able to quit. Don't lose faith in yourself.

> Accept the fact that not everyone can quit "cold turkey." Many people have successfully stopped smoking, all at once, and have never started again. Although this method may work for some people, it does not work for everyone. If you feel that the cold-turkey method is not for you, first, try cutting back on the number of cigarettes, cigars or pipe bowls, you smoke each day. Count the number of cigarettes you smoke in an average day, then smoke one less each day. You may need to count them every morning. Keep a chart and leave out only the number that you

can have that day.

> If you find you cannot stop at this point, switch to a low-tar, low-nicotine brand of cigarettes. But do not increase the *number* of cigarettes you smoke per day. At least you will be making a small step in the right direction.

> Congratulate yourself with each step you take as you eliminate smoking. Giving up smoking is hard. Be proud of yourself *each time* you give up one cigarette.

> According to Merrell Dow Pharmaceuticals Inc., "the risk of smoking again is the highest in the first few months" after you quit. Be careful and reward your achievements. Celebrate your anniversaries of non-smoking. Treat yourself after the first week, the first month and maybe every month after that! You deserve to celebrate!

Pollution: Are you keeping your body in a healthy environment?

Smog, smoking tobacco and breathing tobacco smoke have a significant effect in raising blood pressure.

Death rates, including deaths from heart attacks,

rise when smog attacks a city. The elderly are hit much harder than the younger people, since smog puts a strain on weak hearts and lungs. Carbon monoxide, a component of the pollution from automobile exhuast, can starve the heart of oxygen and even trigger an attack of angina pectoris for those who drive on crowded highways.

Even so, city-wide air pollution is probably a small risk factor when compared with localized pollution from cigarette smoke. Living in the same house with a smoker or working in an office where people smoke puts a person at more risk than living in a city with extremely high air pollution at the peak of the smog season.

Did you know that excessive noise pollution raises blood pressure? It's true. Studies have shown that people who work in noisy environments have lower blood pressure after there is a significant reduction of noise in their environments *(International Archives of Occupational Environmental Health* (59:51-4)*)*.

Chapter Seven

Little-Known Factors in Lowering Blood Pressure

In this chapter we will explore factors that are not generally considered in relation to high blood pressure. We will also give some suggestions for lowering blood pressure that may be new ideas for you to consider.

Your Spouse

Your mother always told you to marry the "right" person, but you probably didn't know how much influence your marriage partner can have on you. The disposition of your spouse or your partner's blood pressure has a great influence on your blood pressure levels. At the University of Texas, Marjorie A. Speers, Ph.D., discovered the relationship after examining over 1,200 couples (*American Journal of*

Epidemiology 123:818-29). Other factors, like exercise, salt intake and obesity were taken into consideration, but the spouse still influenced the blood pressure levels.

Your Pet

Although the doctor may never say, "Take one puppy and call me in the morning," many health professionals are now recommending the loving companionship and responsibility that a pet provides. According to medical studies, in some cases having a pet can help people reduce their high blood pressure levels. Of course, pets aren't for everyone. They require care which some people cannot give.

Your Conversations

Talking too much may irritate your friends, but did you know it could also be hazardous to your health? Studies by James Lynch, Ph.D., of the University of Maryland Medical School show that listening, rather than talking, lowers blood pressure. Most people experience a rise in blood pressure when they speak, followed by a rapid drop when they listen, reports *Arteries Cleaned Out Naturally.* In another report in *Psychosomatic Medicine* (43: 25-33), 98 percent of the 178 people studied had their blood pressure surge when they started talking

The highs and lows of blood pressure level won't hurt people with normal blood pressure, Dr. Lynch explains, but in someone with high blood pressure, the highs can be dangerous.

Dr. Lynch used an automatic blood pressure monitor and recorded continuous blood pressure readings during conversations with patients. In people with high blood pressure, talking about intimate problems raised their blood pressure into the "danger zone," according to Dr. Lynch.

Many people with high blood pressure do not speak normally, which causes their blood pressure to rise even further. Dr. Lynch claims that the louder and faster a person talks, the higher the blood pressure. People who emphasize their words, talk "breathlessly," use hand motions, interrupt or talk over someone else seem to experience the highest blood pressure raises.

Dr. Lynch believes that slower speaking, combined with breathing more deeply and regularly during speech, helps to lower blood pressure. Anyone with speech-induced blood pressure problems can learn to speak more slowly, he says.

Learning to listen and focusing on what the person is saying may lower stress and reduce the load on the heart. Most people with chronic high blood pressure do not really "listen" to a conversation, Lynch explains. These people are so worried about how they will reply that they are defensive even when they are listening and their blood pressure doesn't drop as much as it does in a person who truly listens.

In a University of Pennsylvania study, Drs. Katcher and Beck compared blood pressure levels during three different situations — while the participants just sat and did nothing, while they watched fish in a small tank, and while they talked. The highest level was during speech but the lowest level was while watching the fish. Being quiet isn't the key to lowering your blood pressure. You need to relax and focus on something or someone else. That could be listening to someone talking or it could be caring for a pet or many other activities.

Dr. Lynch believes that the most important thing his studies have shown is that "learning to listen to *other people* can help hypertensives lower their blood pressure."

The next time you visit with your friends or family, listen to what they have to say. It will not only help them, it will also do your own heart good.

Your Medications

Your pharmacist or your doctor can tell you if any prescription drugs you are taking can raise blood pressure. These are some of the drugs known to cause elevate blood pressure: oral contraceptives, Dobutrex Vials®, Proventil Inhaler®, Sandimmune®, Tolectin® 200 and DS Capsules, and Ventolin Inhaler®. Birth control pills were first linked to high blood pressure in 1967 by Dr. John Laragh (*Journal of the American Medical Association* 201: 918:22). Over the years several other studies have verified the suspicions. The longer "The Pill" is used and the older you are when you take it the higher your chances are of developing high blood pressure.

During the first year on oral contraceptives, women should have their blood pressure checked once every two months. If it is elevated, a different form of birth control should be used. Once "The Pill" is stopped, blood pressure should return to a regular level within four months.

There are hundreds of drugs, including over-the-counter diet pills, which list high blood pressure as a side effect, so be sure to read the warnings listed on any non-prescription or prescription medicines you may buy.

Illegal drugs, like cocaine, are also associated with raising blood pressure levels and should be avoided.

Be sure to check with your doctor before discontinuing medicine.

Your Sexual Habits

One of the questions doctors get asked most by men with high blood pressure is "can I still have a regular sex life?" In most cases, patients with high blood pressure can continue their sexual relations with their spouse without any problems. If you do experience unusual symptoms like shortness of breath or chest pain following sex, see your doctor as soon as possible and discuss these problems with him or her.

However, having an affair greatly increases the stress level and the risk of having a heart attack during the sexual relations.

Some drugs prescribed for high blood pressure can cause a reduced sex drive and make it difficult to maintain an erection. However, in a recent study by the University of Connecticut Health Center, Boston University and several other centers, three drugs were compared for their sex-related side effects.

Propranolol and methyldopa were found to cause a decrease in sex drive and made it difficult to maintain an erection, reports the study in *The Archives of Internal Medicine* (148:788-94). Sexual problems were the worst in men over 51 years who were taking methyldopa or propranol and a diuretic. Captopril, the third drug in the study, did not seem to have any affect on either problem, making it the best choice to avoid sexual problems.

Since doctors believe that some men avoid treatment for high blood pressure because they worry about losing their sex drive, this study is very reassuring.

If you are taking prescription drugs for blood pressure and lower sex drive is a problem side effect, be sure to discuss this with your doctor to see if an alternative drug may work better for you.

Breathing Exercises

Daily breathing exercises may help reduce high blood pressure. Practice by lying flat on your back on a carpeted floor. Prop up your head and put a cushion under your knees so you are completely comfortable and relaxed. Breathe in slowly (to the count of ten), hold for two seconds, then breathe out slowly (another count of ten). Many people feel that they are practicing good breathing just by breathing in slowly, but slow exhaling is just as important. By doing these deep breathing exercises for only three to five minutes each day, you will feel relaxed and may lower your blood pressure and pulse rate.

Straining

Avoid holding your breath when straining. This type of straining is called the Valsalva maneuver, and it often occurs during a bowel movement, while exercising or when you are trying to lift, pull, push or move something. Many times, people hold their breath and grunt and groan when straining. However, holding your breath during these strenuous times causes your blood pressure to skyrocket and puts additional pressure on your heart and arteries. Practice breathing in and out slowly and steadily. Consciously breathe during any strenuous activity. Breathe out on the effort and in on the recovery to limit harm to your blood pressure, researchers from Ithaca College suggest.

Avoid all straining during bowel movements. The strain may cause hemorrhoids and bowel problems as well as increasing your blood pressure.

Flotation Centers

A man suffering from hypertension enters what looks like a Porsche without wheels. Actually it is a tank with no windows, filled with densely salted water. When the hatch is closed he lies back and floats effortlessly in the buoyant water, which is heated to body temperature. The tank is pitch dark and soundproof, and he has the feeling of being suspended in time and space. Tensions gently ebb away.

Flotation centers, whether they use a Porsche-like water tank or just an overgrown bathtub in a dark, soundproof room, are becoming the rage, according to *Psychology Today*. An hour session runs from $20 to $30.

Doctors call the treatment Restricted Environmental Stimulation Therapy, or REST. Studies have shown it not only relaxes people but reduces their blood pressure as well.

Neuroendocrinologist John W. Turner, Jr., and clincial psychologist Tomas H. Fine at the Medical College of Ohio found that after 20 flotation sessions a patient's blood pressure was reduced. Hormones related to stress also decreased in most cases, and heart and respiration rates dropped.

Psychology Today cites a study of twenty borderline hypertensives at the State University at Stoney Brook. Blood pressure decreased after floating once or twice a week for just five weeks, according to the study.

REST has also been known to reduce pain in rheumatoid arthritis sufferers. Some research suggests it can even enhance learning ability.

How does it work? No one knows for sure, but Peter Suedfeld of the University of British Columbia has an idea about why it is effective in reducing blood pressure. Suedfeld says it has to do with focus.

By necessity we pay more attention to external information than internal. During REST however, there is no external material to deal with. Instead, attention is "focused on the internally generated material," Suedfeld says.

Turner adds that when the normal bombardment of external stimuli we constantly face is removed, the body adjusts itself to a new, optimal blood pressure "set point."

The bottom line is this: life today is demanding and offers constant external stimulation; we need a break or, as Suedfeld puts it, a "going away." Suedfeld feels the more demanding a society, the greater the need for a period of "going away-ness." REST is just what the doctor orders.

Cancer

Cancer may cause high blood pressure. Several studies have linked high blood pressure and cancer, but a new Canadian study shows that cancer may *cause* high blood pressure. Until now, many researchers believed that high blood pressure increased one's risk of developing cancer. But, the study in the medical journal *Cancer* (59:7,1386) revealed that blood pressure increased due to the cancer, rather than causing the cancer.

Part Three

If Drugs Are Prescribed

If you're taking drugs to control high blood pressure, this part of the book is for you. We want you to know there is much that you can do to help your doctor care for you even if you are already taking medication. First we must emphasize again that you should never stop taking your medication on your own. This can cause very serious problems. Work with your doctor. Let him help you try to become free of the medications and only employ natural methods with his consent. Your doctor will monitor your progress with you and help you alter your prescriptions safely.

One of the most important ways you can work

with your doctor is to learn all you can about the drug or drugs you are taking. Chapter Eight will describe blood pressure drugs. You will understand what the drugs are doing to your body and what possible side effects you might experience. This will help you work with your doctor to find out if you are taking the most effective drug for *you.* Each person is unique, and the only way your doctor can become an expert on your situation is for you to provide him the best feedback you can. Remember, even with their disadvantages, treatment of high blood pressure with drugs is better than leaving it untreated.

Then in Chapter Nine we will give you some tips on taking medication, and draw some conclusions about the use of prescription drugs and lowering blood pressure naturally.

Chapter Eight

A Description of the General Types of Blood Pressure Medications

When your doctor prescribes a drug, it belongs to a general category of drugs. All the drugs in the group act in a similiar way to solve a problem.

Here are some brief descriptions of the major drug groups used to treat high blood pressure. The drugs are listed with the generic (or chemical name) first, followed by the brand names. Remember that many of the drugs can be purchased in generic form as well as by their brand names.

ACE Inhibitors

ACE is an abbreviation for Angiotensin Converting Enzyme. These drugs stop the production of *angiotensin*, a hormone that causes high blood pressure. ACE inhibitors cause the ACE enzyme to "bind" in the body. When the ACE enzyme is not available, blood pressure is maintained at a regular level. This is a new class of drugs that has been introduced in the 1980s.

The problem with these drugs is that ACE inhibition works for a little while, but then the body begins to make more of the angiotensin hormone to adjust for what is lost because of the drug. Eventually the high blood pressure gets worse, unless you continue on higher doses of the prescription drug.

ACE inhibitors should be used with caution by people with poor kidney function, autoimmune disease (like rheumatoid arthritis or lupus), or people on drugs affecting white blood cells or immune response. While on ACE inhibitor treatment, excessive perspiration, dehydration, vomiting, mouth sores, fever, sore throat, swelling of the hands or feet, irregular heartbeat, chest pains, water retention, skin rash, changes in taste, difficulty in breathing, diarrhea, or any signs of infection should be reported to the doctor immediately. Over-the-counter cough, cold or allergy medications should be avoided. Aspirin or indomethacin decreases the effectiveness of captopril and should be avoided. Patients also taking diuretics may experience severe loss of blood pressure during first three hours after receiving the first dose of an ACE inhibitor. ACE inhibitors most frequently prescribed are:

> captopril (Capoten®)
> enalapril (Vasotec®)
> lisinopril (Prinivil®, Zestril®)

Beta Blockers

Your body has a type of built-in alarm system that switches on whenever you face an emergency or any sort of stressful situation. This is called the *emergency nervous system* and it causes you to put forth your best efforts to deal with stressful situations.

If your blood pressure is normal, your alarm system is probably functioning as it is meant to — now and then raising your energy level, your "get up and go," and making you a capable, productive person.

If your blood pressure is high, however, your alarm system may be turned on too much of the time. You may not feel tense, but your nervous system could be too active. This could be an inherited condition or it could result from your life situation. As we mentioned in Chapter Seven, for some people the emergency nervous system can be activated by simple things, like talking.

Beta-adrenergic blocking agents, known as beta blockers, work to keep your emergency nervous system blocked so that your heart will beat more slowly and your blood pressure will fall. They block the action of naturally occurring substances, like norepinephrine and epinephrine, that stimulate the heart. These substances, which are released into the circulation in response to physical exertion or other stress, cause an increase in heart rate and in the force with which the heart pumps blood. By decreasing the rate and force of the heart contraction, beta blockers reduce blood pressure levels.

Beta blockers are generally less effective than thiazide diuretics in treating high blood pressure in blacks. However, thiazide diuretics and beta blockers seem to be about equally effective in treating whites, reports the *Journal of the American Medical Association* (248:1996).

Unfortunately, these drugs may also "block" your enjoyment of life, dulling your energy levels, leaving you drowsy or feeling lethargic most of the time. You may begin to feel like you don't care much about life anymore and chalk it up to just "getting older." Often these feelings come on so gradually that you may not realize that it is the drug that is causing you to feel this way.

Beta blockers should not be used (or be used with great caution) by people with asthma, hay fever or history of congestive heart failure. Beta blockers may interfere with heart activity during major surgery and with the treatment of overactive thyroid, low blood sugar, diabetes, kidney disease or liver disease. Beta blockers may change the effectiveness of insulin, anti-inflammatory drugs, antihistamines and antidiabetic drugs. Avoid alcohol. Alcohol can cause dangerously low blood pressure when combined with a beta blocker. Smoking may reduce the effectiveness of the beta blocker, propranolol.

How much better it would be if you could manage your blood pressure through doctor approved lifestyle changes — like reducing stress through exercise and healthy habits — than to suffer the side effects and expense of these drugs.

However, remember this warning. If you have been taking a beta blocker and suddenly stop, your body may react by raising your blood pressure to *dangerously* high rates. If you want to stop taking medication, you must do it *gradually* and under the watchful care and consent of your doctor as natural methods prove effective. Beta blockers most frequently prescribed are:

> acebutolol (Sectral®)
> atenolol (Tenormin®)
> metoprolol (Lopressor®)
> nadolol (Corgard®)
> pindolol (Visken®)
> propranolol (Inderal®, Inderal® LA)
> timolol (Blocadren®, Timolide®)

Blood Pressure Reducers

These drugs are known as "antihypertensives" and act in a variety of different ways to help lower high blood pressure levels. This is not really a specific class of drugs but a general grouping of several different kinds of drugs.

Guanethidine can cause low blood pressure and a loss of balance when you stand quickly. Drinking alcohol, exercising or hot weather can aggravate this side effect. Diarrhea and sexual problems in men are also common.

People with a history of depression should not take reserpine. Since it can cause severe depression even in someone without depression problems in his past, treatment with reserpine, like all blood pressure reducers, needs to be carefully monitored. Here are some frequently prescribed blood pressure reducers:

> clonidine (Catapres®)
> guanabenz (Wytensin®)
> guanadrel (Hylorel®)
> guanethidine (Ismelin Sulfate®)
> hydralazine (Apresazide®, Ser-Ap-Es®)
> labetalol (Normodyne®, Trandate®)
> methyldopa (Aldomet®)
> minoxidil (Loniten®)
> prazosin (Minipress®)
> rescinnamine (Moderil®)
> reserpine (Demi-Regroton®, Diupres®, Hydromox®, Regroton®, Serpasil®)
> terazosin (Hytrin®)

Calcium Channel Blockers

These medicines interfere with the transport of calcium into the heart and vein muscle cells and inhibit their contraction. This causes the veins and arteries to enlarge and reduce the heart rate and blood pressure. Calcium channel blockers are mostly used in the treatment of angina. However, the calcium channel blocker, verapamil, can also be used in the management of high blood pressure.

Dizziness, lightheadedness, flushing, hot feelings and fluid retention are just some of the side effects of this class. Taking beta blockers at the same time as calcium channel blockers is usually well tolerated, but may cause heart failure in people with aorta problems, who are also taking beta blockers. Don't withdraw suddenly from beta blockers before or during calcium channel blocker therapy. Prescriptions for calcium channel blockers include:

- > diltiazem (Cardizem®)
- > nifedipine (Procardia®)
- > verapamil (Calan®, Isoptin®, Isoptin® SR)

Diuretics

According to a recent Gallup survey, the diuretic Dyazide® is the most commonly recommended high blood pressure drug of any class, with more than twice as many doctors prescribing it than any other diuretic.

Approximately 60 percent of newly-diagnosed hypertension patients are begun on diuretics, according to drug manufacturer Ciba-Geigy. The majority of these people receive thiazide diuretics.

Often called "water pills," diuretics are chemicals which act on the kidneys, causing them to flush salt and water from the body. To understand how these drugs lower blood pressure, you must remember how important our kidneys are to our health. One of the main jobs of our kidneys is to flush out the excess salt and minerals from our bodies each day. However, if over the years we've eaten too much salt or are salt retentive, the kidneys can't take salt out fast enough, and it builds up in our bodies. We then retain extra fluid to dilute the salt.

Our bodies begin to sense a problem—there's too much salt and fluid building up in the system. So to solve the problem our blood pressure rises, forcing the kidneys to flush out the extra salt and fluids.

The function of the diuretics is to help the kidney take out the excess salt and fluid so that our blood pressure doesn't have to rise to do the job. As fluid volume in the blood vessels drops, the blood pressure also goes down.

Diuretics are also prescribed to add to the effectiveness of other blood pressure reducing drugs.

One problem with this type of drug is that it may

be hard to find one that will really work well in your particular body. Either they simply aren't sufficient or they are too potent and make you run to the bathroom continually. To find the right drug at the right dose for you can be very difficult.

Also, if you continue to eat a lot of salt and you are on a diuretic that is flushing it out of your system, the drug will also be flushing out too many other minerals from your body, like potassium. It has been estimated that the majority of patients receiving diuretics exhibit one or more of the signs and symptoms of low potassium. Therefore, potassium supplements are usually prescribed as well, unless the patient is receiving "potassium sparing" diuretics.

Thiazide diuretics should be used with caution by people with poor kidney function or progressive liver disease. Sensitivity reactions are most likely to occur in people with allergies or bronchial asthma. Thiazide diuretics can cause severe sunburn with modest exposure to the sun. Insulin requirements may have to be adjusted. Pain relievers and barbitutrates may cause increased effects of the diuretics and should be avoided if possible. Thiazide diuretics also interact with digitalis and related drugs, adrenocorticoids, and tricyclic antidepressant drugs.

Clearly, the diuretic drugs, though they are very often prescribed, are not without serious drawbacks. One recent study showed that patients with unstable angina who received thiazide diuretics had higher death rates than those who didn't. Commonly prescribed diuretic drugs include:

Thiazide and Similar Diuretics
> bendroflumethiazide (Naturetin®)
> benzthiazide (Exna®, Hydrex®)
> chlorothiazide (Diuril®)
> chlorthalidone (Hygroton®, Thalitone®)
> cyclothiazide (Anhydron®, Fluidil®)
> hydrochlorothiazide (Esidrix®, HydroDIURIL®)
> hydroflumethiazide (Diucardin®, Saluron®)
> indapamide (Lozol®)
> methyclothiazide (Enduron®, Aquatensen®)
> metolazone (Diulo®, Microx®, Zaroxolyn®)
> polythiazide (Renese®)
> quinethazone (Hydromox®)
> trichlormethiazide (Metahydrin®, Naqua®)

Loop Diuretics
> bumetanide (Bumex®)

> ethacrynic acid (Edecrin®)
> furosemide (Lasix®)

Potassium Retaining Diuretics
> amiloride (Midamor®)
> spironolactone (Aldactone®)
> triamterene (Dyrenium®)

Combinations

Combinations of different types of drugs are sometimes used to make it easier for people to remember to take their medication and to have the most efficient use of the drugs in the body. They are not usually given as the initial treatment for high blood pressure, since the individual doses of each drug need to be adjusted separately before the optimum "combination" for each person can be obtained. Here are some combinations that are often prescribed:
> Alazide® (spironolactone and hydrochlorothiazide)
> Aldactazide® (spironolactone and hydrochlorothiazide)
> Capozide® (captopril and hydrochlorothiazide)

> Dyazide® (triamterene and hydrochlorothiazide)
> Lopressor HCT® (metoprolol and hydrochlorothiazide
> Maxzide® (triamterene and hydrochlorothiazide)
> Moduretic® (amiloride and hydrochlorothiazide)
> Normozide® (labetalol and hydrochlorothiazide)
> Spironazide® (spironolactone and hydrochlorothiazide)
> Spirozide® (spironolactone and hydrochlorothiazide)
> Tenoretic® (atenolol and chlorthalidone)
> Unipres® (reserpine, hydralazine, and hydrochlorothiazide)
> Vaseretic® (enalapril and hydrochlorothiazide)

MAO Inhibitors

Another group of drugs that works by inhibiting a normal body action is the monoamine oxidase (MAO) inhibitors. They stop the body from producing certain chemicals in the brain and nerves.

They have many side effects like dizziness and weakness. Lowering blood pressure is really just one more side effect. MAO inhibitors are antidepressant drugs, although pargyline (Eutonyl®) has been used to treat high blood pressure. Since high blood pressure is also a possible side effect of pargyline, and its effects must be closely monitored, the doctors of *The Medical Letter* recommend that this drug should *not* be used in the treatment of high blood pressure.

There are other MAO inhibiting drugs but we have not listed them since they are not used in the treatment of high blood pressure.

Potassium Supplements

Potassium is a mineral that is sometimes needed to offset the side effects of certain blood pressure reducing drugs which lower the body's potassium to below normal levels. Adults need 1525-5625 mg. of potassium daily, according to the U.S. Recommended Dietary Allowance.

While some foods such as bananas, apricots, and raisins contain relatively high amounts of potassium, it is difficult to eat enough to replace the potassium lost through certain drugs. Supplements are often needed because it would not be practical to eat enough potassium-rich foods, says the *New England Journal of Medicine* (313:582-582). It reports that since each inch of an average banana contains approximately 2mEq (milligram equivalents) of potassium . . . and patients taking diuretics require 60-80mEq each day, they would need to eat 2.5-3.3 feet of bananas daily to get enough!

Some medical authorities recommend switching from regular table salt to a type of light salt which is half sodium chloride and half potassium chloride. It would be good advice to seek a medical opinion from a physician before doing this since too much potassium is extremely dangerous.

Potassium supplements should not be used or used only with great caution by people who have kidney disease, impaired kidney function, kidney obstruction or heart disease or who are taking a prescription diuretic that is potassium-retaining, because excessive potassium can be harmful or even fatal. Diabetics and people with severe burns should use this mineral with caution.

Megadoses of potassium should be avoided because high levels of potassium can cause fatal heart attacks. Potassium is often prescribed as follows:

> potassium bicarbonate (K-Lyte®)
> potassium chloride (Kay Ciel®, K-Lor®, Klotrix®, K-Tab®, Micro-K Extencaps®, Micro-K 10®, Slow-K®, Ten-K™)
> potassium gluconate (Kaon®)

The Effectivness of Prescription Drugs

The only truly safe way to help lower your blood pressure is to stop doing what's causing it if you can. If you have practiced all the natural ways we have discussed, and your doctor still feels you need medication, be sure you know and monitor the drug or drugs you are taking so that you can advise your doctor of any side effects. Also, you can help him determine whether any drug is actually doing what it was intended to do.

If you would like more detailed information, drug by drug, on the medications you may be taking for high blood pressure, or other problems, you will enjoy our *Prescription Drug Encyclopedia.* Published by FC&A, this valuable reference explains intended effects, side effects, warnings and dangerous drug interactions of over 700 of the most commonly prescribed drugs. You can order a copy by mailing \$11.97 + \$3.00 postage and handling to: FC&A, 103 Clover Green, Peachtree City, GA 30269.

Chapter Nine

Conclusion: Prescription Drugs and Lowering Blood Pressure Naturally

You've now read all about high blood pressure, you've heard how it can be lowered naturally, and you've also seen the descriptions of the types of medicine you may be taking. Where does this leave you? This chapter will draw some conclusions about your situation and help you come to a point of decision about how you will handle your blood pressure problem.

When is blood pressure medication prescribed?

Drug treatment for mild to moderate high blood pressure has been extremely controversial within the medical profession because doctors are not sure when blood pressure levels are high enough to begin using prescription drugs. A recent study in Sweden found that reducing blood pressure to lower than the level of 150/85 in middle-aged men had no effect on their risk of heart or artery disease. The study (*Journal of the American Medical Association* 259:2553-2557) at the University of Goteberg was conducted over 12 years.

However, another new study has shown that early drug treatment can save lives. People with mild high blood pressure who took drugs had 40 percent fewer fatal strokes and 38 percent fewer non-fatal strokes, in research that Dr. Charles Hennekens recently presented to an American Heart Association meeting in San Francisco. Therefore, treating mild or moderate high blood pressure with drugs may save lives. There continues to be a lot of controversy on the best use of drugs in people with low or moderate hypertension.

In spite of the controversy, high blood pressure is usually treated by physicians with drugs. In a recent Gallup poll, seven in ten patients reported that their doctor prescribed medication immediately upon initial diagnosis of high blood pressure. A study by the Joint National Committee on Detection, Evaluation, and Treatment of High Blood Pressure (*Archives of Internal Medicine* 144: 1045) decided that most people with high blood pressure need drug treatment.

Prescription drugs can have positive benefits. They are easy to prescribe and easy for the patient to take, so they are the most common treatment.

Prescription drugs are often overprescribed because many doctors are reluctant to offer any alternatives to drugs to their patients. Even though prescription drugs may not be the best solution, some patients *demand* a prescription from their doctor so that "their trip to the doctor wasn't wasted." A recent study by the U.S. Social Security Administration revealed that most doctors don't tell their patients about the possible side effects of drugs they prescribe. Ironically, the same study showed that a majority of patients don't follow their doctors' directions for taking the drugs that are prescribed.

Doctors are not always excited about the extended natural treatment of high blood pressure. "The long-term routine care of hypertensive patients offers us no challenge," Dr. Frank Finnerty wrote in an editorial in *The New England Journal of Medicine*. Finnerty believes that doctors are often unconcerned about the effects of high blood pressure because it is a long-term, routine type of problem. Because of this uncaring attititude, non-drug alternatives that require education, commitment and time are often ignored or unmentioned by doctors.

If high blood pressure is diagnosed, your doctor should review your family history and administer some tests to make sure that it hasn't affected any of your vital organs. Your doctor should also test for rare causes of high blood pressure, like kidney problems, Cushing's disease or brain tumors.

A new procedure, involving resting for half an hour, taking the drug captopril and then having a special blood test, will help doctors determine if narrow kidney arteries are causing your blood pressure problems. Narrow arteries leading to one or both kidneys causes high blood pressure in just one to five percent of all high blood pressure cases. But if it's discovered, the cure may be simple — angioplasty.

In angioplasty a balloon-tipped catheter is inserted into the blocked artery leading to the kidney. The balloon is expanded and contracted several times which helps to crush the plaque and widen the blood vessel. Blood pressure was reduced in 90 percent of over 200 patients who had narrow kidney arteries and and were treated by angioplasty, Dr. Heinrich Ingrisch reported from the Bogenhasuen Clinic in Munich, Germany. The success continued as 75 percent had normal blood pressure six months after the angioplasty, and 77 percent maintained normal levels five years after surgery.

Yet, if high blood pressure from kidney/artery malfunctions goes undiagnosed, a person may be needlessly treated for high blood pressure. The new test is available at major medical centers throughout the country.

Your eyes, stomach, blood vessels in the legs, kidney function, heart and nervous system should be checked. A complete blood count including thyroid hormone and renin levels, urinalysis (an analysis of the urine), a chest X-ray, and an electrocardiogram (EKG) may also be needed to determine the damage, if any, to your heart, arteries and kidneys.

High levels of thyroid hormone in the blood may show that an overactive thyroid is causing or aggravating the high blood pressure. High or low levels of renin, a substance produced by the kidneys, can also affect the preferred treatment.

All of these factors will help determine whether or not your doctor will prescribe blood pressure medicine and, if needed, what kind of drug will be best for you.

Drug treatment is quite complex because many people have more than one ailment and need several different drugs. The interaction of those drugs and the actions that the drugs have on the body have to be considered for each person, so drug treatment must be individualized. For example, some people with high blood pressure may also have heart problems or high cholesterol levels which will need to be considered when deciding on the correct medication for that person.

Drugs of First Choice

Since many factors enter into blood pressure control, many different drugs are used for treatment. Usually doctors try the most widely accepted drugs first — drugs that usually work best for most people. However, if these drugs don't control the blood pressure, other drugs that are stronger, more expensive or have more serious side effects are tried.

Diuretic drugs are usually prescribed first because they are effective in many people and are relatively inexpensive. ACE inhibitors and calcium channel blockers can also be used as the first step in drug treatment but these drugs are much more expensive. However, a new Swedish study in the *Journal of the American Medical Association* (259:1976-

1982) has shown that fewer people on a beta blocker died from heart attacks or strokes than people on a diuretic. So even though beta blockers can cost several times as much as diuretics and they have not been considered a "first step" drug, the benefits seem to make beta blockers an acceptable first choice.

Medical Letter consultants suggest that "if a diuretic is not chosen as the initial drug and a second drug is necessary, then a diuretic should be used."

Considering the Cost Factor

One in four patients in a recent Gallup survey said that paying for high blood pressure medications was "somewhat" or "very much" of a problem.

Physicians who fail to consider diuretics first when treating high blood pressure may be helping to "break the bank" on prescription costs, according to experts at a medical symposium sponsored by the Leonard Davis Institute of Health Economics at the University of Pennsylvania.

"Wholesale shift to the newer therapies could add a billion dollars or more annually to national costs for high blood pressure treatment," Dr. William Stason of the Harvard School of Public Health said at the symposium.

Despite the increased cost of the newer medicines, the researchers noted that there is no evidence of added clinical benefit for most patients with mild to moderate uncomplicated high blood pressure.

"Only the small minority of patients whose hypertension cannot be successfully controlled or who are bothered by side effects need to be shifted through a progression of costlier drugs," Dr. Stason explained.

More experienced physicians and those who see a higher number of hypertensive patients are more likely to prescribe diuretics as the drugs of first choice, according to a Gallup survey.

But unless your doctor knows that the cost of your care is an important factor to you, you may receive a prescription for one of the most expensive drugs. In the Gallup poll, "only 30 percent of patients actually spoke to their doctors about the cost of their prescriptions," reported Mark Pauly, Ph.D., of the University of Pennsylvania. However, he cautions, "the notion that more expensive means better simply does not carry over to prescription drugs, and there are many Americans, particularly the elderly on fixed incomes, who sometimes pay a premium for products when their scarce resources could be spent better elsewhere."

What should you know if you are taking medication?

Here are some tips for people taking medicine to control high blood pressure:

> Get your blood pressure checked regularly; it takes only a minute or two. If it is above the normal range (140/90), see your doctor.

> Take your prescribed medicine as directed. Keep doing so because, even if you feel better, your high blood pressure is not cured. Regular dosages are necessary to keep it under control.

> Don't change the dose yourself. You might get too much or not enough medicine. Either way it could be harmful. If you take less of your prescription than your doctor prescribes, you may increase the risk of complications such as stroke or heart attack. If you take more of your medication than you're supposed to, you increase the risk of having side effects from the drug.

> Don't stop taking a drug on your own, even if you feel lightheaded, dizzy, tired, depressed or have trouble sleeping. Your drug can be controlling your blood pressure but may also be giving you these or

other side effects. Notify your doctor immediately when bothersome side effects occur. Many times your doctor will be able to switch you to another drug. Your doctor needs to know how medication is affecting you in order to treat your condition properly.

> If you have questions about your high blood pressure or your prescription, don't ask a friend or relative. Their information or advice may be well-intended but wrong for you. Ask your doctor or pharmacist — they are the people qualified to answer.

> Be sure to tell your your doctor and pharmacist about all prescription drugs, any daily vitamin or mineral supplements, or nonprescription drugs (aspirin, cold medicines, laxatives) that you take regularly. Many drugs interact with each other and lose or gain potency or cause serious side effects when taken together.

> Use only one pharmacy, preferably a pharmacy with computerized patient profiles because it has the ability to spot allergic reactions and interactions between medicines. If you have more than one doctor (general and heart specialist, for example), using only one pharmacy will help you keep track of all prescriptions. Then your pharmacy will double-

check that you will take your prescription and non-prescription medication safely.

> Record any side effects you may experience while taking prescription drugs, and report them to your doctor.

> Always follow label instructions. If there is a difference between your doctor's verbal instructions and the label instructions, contact your doctor immediately. If you don't follow the doctor's specific instructions, your medicine may be ineffective or harmful to you.

> *Never* take drugs prescribed for someone else. Drugs should be prescribed after considering other drugs being taken, one's age, weight, health history and other important factors. Exchanging medicine is dangerous; don't do it!

> The National Council on Patient Information and Education says that people ask too few questions about the drugs their doctors prescribe. If you learn more about your prescriptions, you can understand why you should take your drugs properly so they will be most effective. If you are well-informed about your treatment and condition you will know if something unusual occurs, and you will know when to contact your doctor for help. Do not be afraid to write

down your doctor's answers to these questions so you can refer to them later.

- What is the name of the drug?
- What is it supposed to do?
- How long will it take before it is effective?
- How am I supposed to take it?
- When am I supposed to take it?
- Are there any foods, drinks, other drugs or activities that I should avoid while taking this drug?
- What are the drug's side effects?
- What should I do if the side effects happen to me?
- Is written information available on this drug that I could have and understand?
- How can I get this written information?

> Keep a list of all your current prescriptions in your wallet, billfold or purse. Include the name of the drug, what dose you are taking and the name of the doctor who prescribed it. When you visit your doctor (or doctors) have them check your list and keep it up to date. The list will remind them of your current prescriptions, and keeping it with you could help

avoid dangerous drug interactions. During an emergency, the list will provide valuable information at the attending doctor's fingertips.

> Some companies are now producing small cards, the size of credit cards, that contain a computer chip listing your important health information including current medical evalution, normal blood pressure, heart readings, and current prescriptions. In case of an emergency, the card could provide important information, and save your life. Ask your doctor or pharmacist how you can get one of these cards.

> Ibuprofen, an over-the-counter pain reliever, may interfere with prescription drugs controlling blood pressure, according to research by the University of Cincinnati Medical Center (*Annals of Internal Medicine*). Blood pressure levels increased about seven points in just three weeks in patients who took ibuprofen for pain while receiving blood pressure medicine. Increased blood pressure did not occur when aspirin or acetaminophen was used for pain, the study reports.

Ibuprofen is found in many over-the-counter medicines for pain and menstrual cramps including Advil®, Haltran®, Ibuprin®, Medipren®, Nuprin®, Pamprin-IB® and Trendar®. Ibuprofen in prescription strengths, used mostly for the pain of arthritis, is available as Ifen®, Motrin®, and Rufen®. The doctors in the study suggest that patients taking any type of blood pressure medicine should refrain from using ibuprofen.

> Inderal® and other beta-blocking drugs, prescribed to help lower high blood pressure, may cause depression, according to a study in the *Journal of the American Medical Association* (255:357-360). More than 20 percent of people taking beta-blockers eventually start taking antidepressant drugs, says Dr. Jerry Avorn of Harvard Medical School, who conducted the study. Dr. Avorn says this is the first study that linked depression and beta-blockers, although many doctors have suspected a connection for several years. If you suspect your blood pressure medication is causing depression, discuss alternatives with your doctor. Never stop taking a prescribed drug without your doctor's consent.

> Even if you are taking a prescription drug, with your doctor's knowledge, you should still try to reduce your salt, improve your diet, get regular exercise and do all the things you can to help lower your blood pressure naturally. These changes will enable your doctor to prescribe the least amount medication

possible. A recent study at the Indiana University School of Medicine, found that one-third of people who cut back on sodium were able to reduce their blood pressure and their medication (*Journal of the American Medical Association* 259:2561-5).

What are the disadvantages of blood pressure medications?

Blood pressure drugs can cause miserable side effects like headaches, poor appetite, upset stomach, dry mouth, diarrhea, stuffy nose, tingling or numbness in hands or feet, dizziness, cramps, depression, rashes, chills, fever, constipation, aching joints, difficult urination or low sex drive.

A study reported in the *Journal of the American Medical Association* (253:3263-68) involving 3,844 patients with high blood pressure found that 9.3 percent of them stopped drug treatment because of "definite" or "probable" side effects, and an additional 23.4 percent stopped drug treatment because of "possible" side effects.

Drug treatment is only effective when the drugs are taken as prescribed. Since high blood pressure is not felt, many people stop taking their medication because "they are feeling fine." About half of the high blood pressure patients in a 1973 Harris poll quit taking their prescription because "they thought they were cured." This can lead to dangerously high blood pressure levels. Never stop taking or change anything about your prescribed medication without your doctor's knowledge and consent.

Other people forget to take their prescriptions or have difficulty affording prescription drugs over long periods of time. These are serious drawbacks and concerns about relying on prescription drugs for complete control of blood pressure.

Of an estimated 58 million Americans with high blood pressure, about 19 million are currently being treated with available medications. According to a survey by the Joint National Committee on Detection, Evaluation, and Treatment of High Blood Pressure, only one-third of the patients taking medication actually have their blood pressure under satisfactory control.

High blood pressure *can* often be lowered without drugs. For example, in one recent university test, 85.3 percent of patients with high blood pressure were able to quit taking their medication. Even without drugs, their blood pressures remained lower than when they were on drugs. The hundreds of people in the study also found that their blood cholesterol levels dropped 26 percent. The doctor in charge of the program said, "You lose your tiredness. You feel much more active. You have a general feeling of well being."

The people in this study lowered their blood pressure by making changes in their lifestyles involving nutrition and moderate exercise, as described in Part Two of this book.

Remember that high blood pressure is not "cured" but it can be controlled. Learning to control your blood pressure is a lifelong committment. If you and your doctor choose non-drug methods, they must be continued for the rest of your life, just as prescription drugs would be.

Choosing just one area, like salt reduction, and concentrating on it, may not help lower your blood pressure. It is the effective combination of natural methods that will give you the best results. For example, many people try exercising or eating a low-sodium, high-potassium diet. In a recent study by James Mitchell, Ph.D., in *Psychosomatic Medicine*, people lost about ten points diastolic on either a diet or exercising. But when they combined diet and exercise they lowered their blood pressure an additional four points.

The first step you should take to lower your blood pressure naturally is to talk with your doctor about the methods we've described. Have your doctor monitor your blood pressure levels as you gradually make changes in your diet and lifestyle. Your doctor will probably be as excited as you are when your body gradually needs less and less of the medication. Perhaps he will even help you celebrate when you finally reach your goal of independence from your medicine cabinet and freedom from the side effects of prescription blood pressure drugs.

Dr. Cleaves M. Bennett, author of *Control Your High Blood Presssure Without Drugs*, says:

"In the years since I stopped always prescribing pills for high blood presssure and started treating it with an emphasis on diet and exercise and relaxation, I've seen a different look on my patients' faces.

"I have seen them happier, more assured, and younger-looking. I have seen people coming into my office looking and feeling healthier than they have in years. I have seen that what I am doing has made a difference in their lives. That look in their eyes, if you ask me, is what (practicing) medicine is all about."

That, too, is what this book has been all about. To help you further we have prepared "A Treasury of Helps" at the end of this book for your reference.

Part Four

A Treasury of Helps

Appendix One

Blood Pressure Chart

Record your blood pressure every time it is measured, even when taken by your doctor. Keep a chart like this with you in case of an emergency and show it to your doctor at office visits.

Date	Time	Reading	Arm
		/	
		/	
		/	
		/	
		/	

Appendix Two

Fourteen Day Menus

Daily Menus

The menus that follow recommend foods that are low in cholesterol fat, salt and calories and high in fiber. Check with your doctor before you use this plan. If your doctor doesn't want you to lose weight, you should increase the size of each food portion. Or even better, eat small meals and small between-meal snacks of foods from the "good" list. The foods that are underlined are included in the recipe section (Appendix Three). All soups should be homemade without salt.

First Day

Breakfast: 1 cup of 5-minute oatmeal with skimmed milk, sweetened with bananas or raisins
1 small glass of unsweetened orange juice
1 piece of whole wheat toast (sweeten with one teaspoon of honey — no butter)
Water, decaffeinated coffee, tea or skimmed milk

Lunch: Large sliced chicken sandwich on whole wheat bread (no mayonnaise or butter)
Lettuce, tomato and bean salad (make your own oil-free dressing with vinegar, water and seasoning)
Fresh fruit cocktail (1/2 cup)
Water

Dinner: 3 ounces of broiled veal
1 piece of bran bread toast
1 cup of green beans

1 cup of brown rice
1 bowl of green salad
Water, decaffeinated coffee, or tea

Second Day

Breakfast: 3 pieces of cinnamon toast with 1 teaspoon honey for each piece (use whole wheat or homemade bran bread — no butter)
1 glass of unsweetened orange juice
Water, decaffeinated coffee, or tea

Lunch: 1 bran muffin
1 tuna salad sandwich on whole wheat or bran bread
1 apple with peel
Skimmed milk

Dinner: 1 serving of cod and rice bake
1/2 cup of lima beans
1/2 unsweetened peach
Water, decaffeinated coffee, or tea

Third Day

Breakfast: 3 slices of whole wheat or homemade bran bread — (no butter)
1/2 fresh unsweetened grapefruit
Water, decaffeinated coffee, tea or skimmed milk

Lunch: Cottage cheese salad (1 cup of 1% low-fat cottage cheese on a lettuce leaf surrounded by 1 sliced tomato and kidney beans marinated in vinegar)
2 ounces of low-fat American cheese on bran bread (read the labels to find a cheese with 1/2 the calories and 1/3 the fat of regular cheese)
Water

Dinner: 3 ounces of meatloaf
1 baked potato (no butter)
1 cup of stewed tomatoes
1 dinner roll
Water, decaffeinated coffee, or tea

Fourth Day

Breakfast: 2 bran muffins (no butter)
1 glass of unsweetened orange juice
Water, decaffeinated coffee, or tea

Lunch: Sliced turkey sandwich on whole wheat or bran bread
1 raw carrot
Skimmed milk

Dinner: 3 ounces broiled ground beef patty
1 cup tomato soup (low sodium/homemade)
2 dinner rolls
1 bowl of kidney bean or three bean salad
1 brownie
Water, decaffeinated coffee, or tea

Fifth Day

Breakfast: 3 ounces broiled trout or cod
1 piece whole wheat or bran bread toast
1 prune

Water, decaffeinated coffee, or tea

Lunch: Grilled cheese sandwich on whole wheat or bran bread (Use 2 ounces of low-fat American cheese and grill without butter in a non-stick pan.)
1 cup homemade vegetable soup
1 bran muffin
Water

Dinner: 3/4 cup tuna salad
1 dinner roll
1/2 cup easy cooked beets
1 brownie
Water, decaffeinated coffee, or tea

Sixth Day

Breakfast: 1 bowl of oatmeal
1 glass of unsweetened fruit juice
Water, decaffeinated coffee, or tea

Lunch: 1 1/2 cups of brown rice
1 cup unsweetened fruit cocktail
1 dinner roll

1 cup green beans
Water

Dinner: 3/4 cup macaroni and cheese (preferably use stone ground whole wheat macaroni available in health food stores)
1 ear of boiled corn on the cob
1 dinner roll
Water, decaffeinated coffee, tea or skimmed milk

Seventh Day

Breakfast: 1 large bowl of oatmeal with banana
1 glass of unsweetened pineapple juice
Water, decaffeinated coffee, or tea

Lunch: 1 tuna salad sandwich on whole wheat or bran bread
1 cup fresh fruit salad
Skimmed milk

Dinner: 3 ounces roast beef
2 roasted potatoes

1 dinner roll
1/2 cup cooked carrots
1 brownie
Water, decaffeinated coffee, or tea

Eighth Day

Breakfast: 1 bowl whole grain cereal with 1 cup unsweetened strawberries
Water, decaffeinated coffee, tea or skimmed milk

Lunch: Grilled cheese sandwich on whole wheat or bran bread
1 cup homemade vegetable soup
Water

Dinner: 4 ounces broiled veal
1/2 cup white acre peas
1 cup broccoli
2 slices whole wheat or bran bread
Water, decaffeinated coffee, or tea

Ninth Day

Breakfast: 2 bowls unsweetened whole grain cereal with skimmed milk
1 piece unsweetened fresh citrus fruit
Water, decaffeinated coffee, or tea

Lunch: 1 cup field peas
1 cup stewed tomatoes
Whole grain crackers (check label to make sure that crackers are low in fat, salt and sugar)
Skimmed milk

Dinner: 1 large piece baked chicken (moisten in skim milk and dip in seasoned cornmeal and bake)
1 baked potato
1 cup steamed carrots
Water, decaffeinated coffee, or tea

Tenth Day

Breakfast: 1 bowl oatmeal with sliced bananas and skimmed milk

1 piece of whole wheat toast or bran bread
Water, decaffeinated coffee, or tea

Lunch: 1 cup macaroni and cheese
Whole grain crackers
Water

Dinner: 1 lean lamb chop
1 cup collard greens
1 baked sweet potato
1 piece cornbread (made without shortening from 100% stone ground whole kernel yellow corn meal)
1/2 unsweetened peach
Water, decaffeinated coffee, or tea

Eleventh Day

Breakfast: 1 bowl whole grain cereal with 1 cup unsweetened strawberries
1 piece whole wheat toast or bran bread
Water, decaffeinated coffee, or tea

Lunch: 1 large slice pita bread

1 cup homemade bean soup
Skimmed milk

Dinner: 5 ounces broiled fish
1 cup new potatoes
1 cup asparagus
1 dinner roll
Water, decaffeinated coffee, or tea

Twelfth Day

Breakfast: 2 bran muffins
1/2 fresh unsweetened grapefruit
Water, decaffeinated coffee, or tea

Lunch: Tuna sandwich on whole wheat or bran bread
1 cup rice pudding
Water

Dinner: 3/4 cup whole wheat macaroni and cheese
1 cup green beans
1 dinner roll
Water, decaffeinated coffee, or tea

Thirteenth Day

Breakfast: 1 cup of 5-minute oatmeal with skimmed milk, sweetened with bananas or raisins
1 bran muffin
1 glass of unsweetened orange juice
Water, decaffeinated coffee, or tea

Lunch: Sliced chicken sandwich on whole wheat or bran bread
1 cup kidney bean salad
1 apple with peel
Skimmed milk

Dinner: 1 serving of cod and rice bake
1/2 cup easy cooked beets
1 large piece whole wheat or bran bread
1 brownie
Water, decaffeinated coffee, or tea

Fourteenth Day

Breakfast: 3 pieces of cinnamon toast on whole wheat or bran bread (with 1 teaspoon

honey for each piece)
1 glass of unsweetened orange juice
Water, decaffeinated coffee, or tea

Lunch: Grilled cheese sandwich on whole wheat or bran bread
1 cup homemade vegetable soup
1 brownie
Water

Dinner: 3 ounces of meat loaf
1 baked potato (with skin — no butter)
1 cup broccoli
2 slices whole wheat or bran bread
Water, decaffeinated coffee, tea or skimmed milk

Appendix Three

Healthful Recipes

Bean Croquettes

2 cups red kidney beans, cooked
1 cup split peas, cooked
1 cup lentils, cooked
1/4 cup soy grits
1/2 cup homemade chicken stock
1/4 tsp. ground fresh pepper
2 egg whites, beaten
2 tablespoons skim milk
1 cup whole wheat bread crumbs
(seasoned and finely rolled)

Mix beans, peas, and lentils and then puree. Combine with grits and seasonings. Add chicken stock. Shape into croquettes. Combine beaten egg whites and skim milk. Dip croquettes in egg mixture and roll in seasoned bread crumbs. Place under a broiler, turning until all sides are brown. Serve hot.

Beans With Onions

1 lb. dried kidney beans
2 ripe tomatoes, quartered
2 cups diced onion
1 cup diced green pepper
chili powder to taste

Follow instructions on the kidney bean package but do not add salt. When all steps have been completed, except for simmering, add tomatoes, onions and chili powder. Simmer for an additional 1 to 2 hours or until beans are done.

Beans, Refried

1 cup dried pinto, kidney or black beans
3/4 cup diced onion
3 cloves garlic
oregano
pepper

Follow cooking instructions on the bean package but do not add salt. Add onion and garlic before simmering. When beans are done (they should be soft and split), drain and season lightly with oregano and pepper. Mash the beans and cook over medium heat in a non-stick skillet until beans begin to dry out. Serve hot.

Beef Stew

2 chopped onions
2 lbs. of extra lean stew meat
5 diced carrots
8 cubed potatoes (leave the skins on)
1 cup of corn

Brown the meat and onion in a non-stick skillet. Add water and simmer for 2 hours. Add other ingredients and simmer for another hour.

Beet and Cucumber Salad, Tossed

8 to 10 large lettuce leaves
1 large cooked beet
1/2 large cucumber

Tear lettuce leaves into small pieces. Wash cucumber well and dice unpeeled. Dice beet and toss with cucumber and lettuce.

Beets, Easy Cooked

1 lb. beets, peeled and grated
1 teaspoon lemon juice
2 1/2 tablespoons water

Place all ingredients in a non-stick frying pan. Cover and cook over medium heat for 10 minutes. Serve hot.

Bran Bread and Dinner Rolls

1/2 cup warm water
2 packages dry active yeast
2 1/2 cups skimmed milk
1/2 cup honey
2 egg whites
9 cups of stone ground whole wheat flour
1 cup of unprocessed bran (see note)

Let yeast stand in slightly warm, but not hot, water for 5 minutes. Boil milk and then add honey. After 15 minutes of cooling, put into mixing bowl with egg whites, yeast and 2 cups of flour. Stir or beat and add bran. Add rest of flour gradually as you knead the dough for 1/2 hour. If dough is still sticky, knead in more flour. Place dough in a bowl and let rise for 1 hour and 45 minutes. Then put in 3 or 4 non-stick loaf pans or roll pans. Let rise again for 1 hour. Bake loaves for about 40 minutes at 350°. Bake rolls for 10 minutes at 425°.

(Note: Pure, unprocessed bran is different from 100% bran cereal. You can use either type in these recipes, but the texture will be slightly different.)

Bran Muffins

1/2 cup warm water
1 1/2 packages dry active yeast
2 1/4 cups skimmed milk
3 tablespoons honey
1/2 cup dark molasses
1 1/2 cup pure unprocessed bran
2 cups whole wheat flour
1 egg white

Heat milk until scalding, then add honey and molasses. Let milk mixture cool (at least 15 minutes so you don't kill the yeast), then add the bran. Add yeast to warm water and set aside for five minutes. Add yeast and wheat flour to bran mixture. Beat the egg white and fold into the batter. Let stand in a warm place for

30 minutes.

Spoon into non-stick muffin tins, filling them 2/3's full. Bake at 350° for 20 to 25 minutes. Makes 2 dozen muffins. One-half cup of raisins or other dried fruit can be added for variety.

Brown Rice

1) Wash the rice by pouring cold water over two cups of brown rice until any dust rises to the surface of the water. Pour off water, and repeat if necessary.

2) Add 3 cups of water to the clean rice and bring to a boil.

3) Cover pot and boil slowly for 45 minutes or until all water is absorbed.

4) Turn off heat and let steam for 10 minutes.

5) Keep the rice in the refrigerator and reheat at mealtime. It can also be frozen and reheated with success.

Brownies

2 egg whites
1/2 cup honey
3/4 cup whole wheat flour

1/3 cup unprocessed bran
1/4 cup safflower or corn oil
1/4 cup cocoa (or carob to be caffeine-free) mixed with 2/3 cup lukewarm water
1 cup chopped pecans
1 teaspoon vanilla

Beat egg whites until stiff. Mix honey, oil, cocoa (mixed with water) and vanilla together. Sift flour, stir with bran into liquid ingredients. Add nuts. Fold egg whites into batter. Bake in a medium sized, greased pan for 35 minutes in a preheated oven at 350°.

Chili

1 lb. bean curd
4 cups fresh ripe tomotoes
10 cups cooked red kidney beans with liquid
2 large chopped onions
1 teaspoon chili powder
1 teaspoon cumin seed
1 clove of garlic

Combine all ingredients in a large heavy pot. Let simmer for 2 to 3 hours.

Cod, Baked

2 lbs. cod fish fillets or a whole codfish
paprika
sage
1/4 cup stock (fish, beef or chicken)
6 tablespoons white wine

Place cod in shallow non-stick baking dish. Combine stock, wine, paprika and sage. Pour over cod and bake in a 350° oven until tender (between 8 to 10 minutes). Serve hot, garnished with chopped parsley.

Cod and Rice Bake

1 lb. chopped cod or other fish
3 stalks sliced celery
1 chopped onion
2 cups stewed tomatoes
1 cup uncooked washed brown rice
1 1/2 cups homemade or low-salt mushroom soup

Preheat oven to 325°. Mix together above ingredients and bake for one hour and 20 minutes in a covered teflon casserole dish. Use 1 1/2 cups per serving.

Corn Pudding

6 ears corn (fresh or frozen)
3 egg whites plus 1 egg yolk
1 cup skim milk
3 tsp. whole wheat flour
dash cayenne pepper

Steam corn for 8-10 minutes. Let cool and cut the corn from the cobs. In a large bowl combine the corn with the skim milk. Beat the eggs and add to the mixture. Then add whole wheat flour and seasonings. Place in a lightly greased casserole dish. Put the dish in a shallow pan filled with water (about 1 inch of water is sufficient). Bake for 30-40 minutes at 400° or until a knife blade comes out dry.

Cottage Cheese Salad

2 cups low-fat cottage cheese
1 small cucumber
1 medium tomato, diced
2 green onions, finely chopped
4 lettuce leaves
pepper
paprika

Wash cucumber well and dice. Do not peel. Mix cottage cheese, diced cucumber, tomato and green onion. Add pepper to taste. Serve on a lettuce leaf and sprinkle with paprika. Serves 4.

Granola Crunch

4 cups of rolled oats
2/3 cup chopped almonds or walnuts
1/2 cup wheat germ
1/2 cup powdered milk
1/4 cup skimmed milk
1/4 cup honey
2/3 cup raisins or other dried fruit

Combine all dry ingredients except the raisins; then combine and stir wet ingredients, and finally mix together. Spread and bake on cookie sheet for 25 minutes at 275°. Stir every 5 minutes. Remove and add raisins. Makes 20 servings.

Gourmet Green Salad

4 large lettuce leaves
2 small yellow squash
1 stalk broccoli

1/2 cup bean sprouts
1/2 cup chick peas (garbanzo beans)
1/2 cup fresh mushrooms
1 medium tomato

Tear lettuce into small pieces. Dice squash, broccoli, tomatoes and mushrooms into small pieces. Toss all ingredients together. Marinate in vinegar, olive oil and spice dressing.

Haddock, Sautéed

2 lbs. haddock fillets cut into 4-inch strips
2 cups cornmeal
paprika
1/4 teaspoon basil
1/8 teaspoon fresh ground pepper
juice of 2 lemons

Brush fillets in lemon juice. Roll the cut up fillets in corn meal which has been seasoned with paprika, basil and pepper. Place the coated fillets in a hot, non-stick skillet. Reduce the heat slightly and cook from 3 to 5 minutes until done.

Kidney Bean Salad

1 lb. cooked kidney beans, drained
1 medium sweet Spanish onion, diced
1/2 medium bell pepper, diced
2 tender celery stalks, diced
1/4 cup seasoned vinegar
1 tablespoon olive oil

Combine all ingredients and chill. Best if left overnight in refrigerator before serving.

Macaroni and Cheese

1/2 lb. macaroni (whole wheat is best)
1 cup low-fat ricotta cheese
1/8 teaspoon cayenne pepper
1 egg white
1/2 cup bread crumbs

Boil macaroni in water for 20 minutes. Blanch in cold water. Layer macaroni and cheese beginning with macaroni and ending with cheese. Pepper first layer of macaroni. Mix other ingredients together and pour over top of dish. Cover with bread crubs. Bake at 350° until top is browned.

Meatloaf

2 lbs. ground lean veal or beef
1 cup bread crumbs
1/4 cup unprocessed bran
1 1/4 cups skimmed milk
1 stalk finely chopped celery
2 beaten egg whites
1/4 cup chopped onion
1 pinch each of: pepper, mustard powder,
sage and garlic

Shape ingredients into a loaf and top with 4 tablespoons tomato paste or low-salt tomato sauce. Bake 1 1/2 hours at 350°.

Okra Supreme

2 lbs. young tender okra
4 large tomatoes, chopped
2 cloves garlic, minced
1 teaspoon crushed oregano
fresh ground pepper
juice of one lemon
1/4 to 1/2 cup salt-free tomato juice

Steam okra for 10 to 15 minutes or until tender. Place

several tablespoons of water in a large fry pan. Using high heat, pan fry garlic and onions. Add tomatoes, okra, and tomato juice. Season with black pepper and oregano. Cover and let simmer for 15 minutes. Cover with lemon juice. Serve hot.

Peppers Stuffed With Corn

6 medium bell peppers
3 cups cooked corn, cut from the cob
1 cup diced fresh tomato
1 very small onion, diced
1/4 tsp. ground black pepper
1 clove garlic, pressed
1 teaspoon chili powder
3 tablespoons whole wheat flour
1 tablespoon vinegar

Remove tops from green peppers, then remove seeds and inside membrane. Parboil in covered saucepan for 5 minutes with vinegar added to the water. Combine remaining ingredients and spoon mixture into bell peppers. Place in baking dish and bake at 375° for 35 minutes or until done.

Ratatouille

1 eggplant
3 zucchini
1 large onion
2 large tomatoes
1 clove garlic
1/2 teaspoon basil
2 tablespoons olive oil
whole wheat bread crumbs

Peel eggplant if skin is tough; otherwise wash and cut into 1/2 inch slices. Slice zucchini, onion and tomatoes. Layer eggplant, onion, zucchini and tomatoes. Mix seasoning with olive oil and pour over the casserole. Bake covered for 30 to 40 minutes at 350° or until vegetables are tender. Put whole wheat bread crubs on top and brown.

Rice Pudding

2 cups uncooked brown rice
4 cups skimmed milk
1/2 cup honey
2 teaspoons vanilla
2 egg whites

1/4 teaspoon cream of tartar

1/4 teaspoon nutmeg

Cook unsalted brown rice according to previous directions, but do not allow to steam at the end. Beat egg whites and cream of tartar until fluffy. Mix slightly undercooked brown rice, beaten egg whites, milk, honey, vanilla, and nutmeg together. Bake in a non-stick pan or casserole dish at 350° for 1 hour. Makes 10 servings.

Salmon, Stuffed

4 salmon fillets

1 1/2 cups soft whole wheat bread crumbs

1/4 cup celery, chopped

1 teaspoon grated onion

1 teaspoon chopped parsley

1/4 teaspoon tarragon

2 teaspoons of olive oil

juice of 1 lemon

1 lemon, sliced

Cut the fillets lengthwise in two pieces and sprinkle with paprika. Combine bread crumbs, celery, onion, parsley and tarragon with the olive oil. Place mixture on fish fillets and roll them around the mixture.

Secure the rolls in place with toothpicks and brush with lemon juice. Place in a 375° oven for 30 minutes. Serve hot.

Slaw

4 cups shredded raw cabbage
1 tablespoon olive oil
1 teaspoon grated onion
1/2 cup seasoned vinegar

Mix cabbage and oil until cabbage is coated with oil. Add onion and toss to combine thoroughly. Add seasoned vinegar, mix and serve.

Spinach Salad

1 lb. fresh spinach
2 1/2 tablespoons lemon juice
1/2 cup sliced mushrooms (preferably fresh)
1/3 cup grated raw carrots
1 1/2 tablespoons olive oil
1/4 teaspoon tamari

Wash spinach thoroughly, removing stems and drain. Combine remaining ingredients in a cup. Pour mixture over the spinach, tossing thoroughly to coat.

Serves 6.

Squash, Stuffed Yellow

8 crookneck squash
2 egg whites, beaten
1 garlic clove, pressed
1 medium onion, chopped
2 tablespoons chopped parsley
1 teaspoon ground basil
1/2 teaspoon ground savory
1 teaspoon olive oil
1 cup whole wheat bread crumbs

Sauté garlic and onion in 2 tablespoons water until onion is clear. Trim squash, cut in half lengthwise and spoon out centers. Add squash centers and seasonings to non-stick fry pan and cook with olive oil until tender. Remove from heat. Add egg whites to squash mixture. Fill raw squash halves with seasoned squash mixture. Sprinkle bread crumbs on top. Bake at 350° for 40 minutes or until tender. Serve hot.

Squash, Summer

3 lb. small yellow squash, diced

3 medium onions, chopped
1 teaspoon allspice
garlic juice

Sauté onions in non-stick fry pan with several teaspoons water mixed with a drop of garlic juice until onions are clear. Add squash and simmer for 15 minutes, stirring occasionally. Season to taste. Serve hot.

Three Bean Salad

1 lb. green beans, drained (fresh cooked)
1 lb. wax beans (fresh cooked)
1 lb. kidney beans (dried and cooked)
1 medium onion, sliced
1 small bell pepper, sliced
1/4 cup olive oil
1/2 tsp. paprika

Combine beans, onion and bell pepper. Combine all other ingredients in a cup and mix well. Pour the seasoned oil over the bean mixture and toss well. Chill overnight.

Tomato Rice

1 1/2 cups brown rice, uncooked
1 1/4 cups water
1 1/4 cups unsalted tomato juice
3/4 cup chopped celery

Bring water and tomato juice to a boil. Slowly add brown rice and celery. Cover and cook over low heat for 40-50 minutes, stirring occasionally. Remove cover during last 5 minutes of cooking.

Trout, Broiled

2 lbs. trout fillets
2 cups fine whole wheat bread crumbs
juice of 2 lemons
1 lemon, sliced
paprika
1/8 teaspoon sage
chopped parsley

Place fillets in shallow baking pan. Brush with the lemon juice and cover with bread crumbs. Sprinkle with sage and paprika. Cook on the top rack of a 400° oven for 20 to 30 minutes. Serve with lemon slices and parsley. Serves 4.

Tuna Salad

4 small lettuce leaves
1 can tuna (7 oz. water packed)
2 hard cooked egg whites, grated
1/2 small onion, grated
2 stalks celery, diced
1 teaspoon lemon juice

Drain tuna. Mix in celery and egg whites. Grate onion and add to mixture. Season with lemon juice. Serve on a lettuce leaf. Serves 4.

Tuna Salad, Tossed

1 medium head of lettuce
3 hard cooked egg whites, grated
2 green onions, diced
1 medium tomato, finely diced
1 can tuna (7 oz. water packed)
2 tablespoons fine bran
pepper
paprika

Tear lettuce into small pieces. Drain tuna and toss with lettuce. Add remaining ingredients and toss well. Add pepper to taste. Sprinkle lightly with paprika.

Vegetable and Fruit Tossed Salad

1 small head of lettuce
1/2 cup orange sections
1/2 cup raw broccoli, chopped coarsely
2 green onions, finely chopped

Tear lettuce into small pieces. Add remaining ingredients and toss well.

Vegetable Delight

2 lbs. fresh vegetables (use oven baked okra, squash, green tomatoes, and asparagus or your favorite)
2 egg whites
1/8 teaspoon freshly ground pepper
2 tablespoons finely chopped parsley
2 tablespoons unprocessed miller's bran

Wash and trim vegetables as individually required. Mix bran with parsley and pepper. Dip vegetables in beaten egg whites and then in bran mixture. Place on non-stick cookie sheet and bake for 15 to 20 minutes or until brown. Serve hot.

Vegetable Salad, Marinated

1 cup whole string beans (fresh cooked)
1/3 cup mushrooms (preferably fresh)
1 small head of cauliflower
1 small Spanish onion, sliced thin
2 small carrots, sliced
4 stalks celery, diced
1/3 cup vinegar
1/3 cup olive oil
1/2 teaspoon pepper

Combine all ingredients. Toss well. Let stand 24 hours in the refrigerator. Mix occasionally. Serve cold.

Yams, Baked

4 large yams, unpeeled and uncooked
1/4 teaspoon nutmeg
1/4 teaspoon cinnamon

Bake yams at 450° in aluminum foil for about 1 hour (until fork tender). Slice yams in half lengthwise when done. Sprinkle spices over yams and serve hot.

Glossary

aneurysm — an abnormal weakness in the wall of a blood vessel, usually an artery, that leads to ballooning. It is most often found in the aorta, which is the biggest artery in the body going from the heart through the chest and abdomen. An aneurysm can swell, enlarge, and eventually rupture.

angina pectoris — a sudden pain or pressure in the chest behind the breastbone which may radiate down the shoulder, neck, arm, hand or back, usually or mainly on the left side of the body. People with angina pectoris may also feel its sensations as burning, choking, or indigestion. It is associated with insufficient blood flowing through narrowed coronary arteries which supply the heart muscle.

angiotensin — a hormone in the blood that raises blood pressure.

arteriosclerosis — artery disease characterized by a loss of artery elasticity, deposits in the arteries, and hardening of the walls of the arteries leading to a decreased blood flow.

artery — any blood vessel that carries blood away from the heart to the various organs and tissues of the body.

atheromas — small raised plaques of mushy cholesterol, fat and foam cells on the inner walls of the arteries.

atherosclerosis — the deposit of cholesterol and other fatty, waxy substances on the inner walls of the arteries, often leading to narrowing and "hardening" of the arteries as scar tissue and calcification form.

blood pressure — the force exerted on the walls of arteries, veins and capillaries as the heart pumps blood through the body.

capillaries — minute blood vessels that connect the smallest arteries to the smallest veins.

cardiac — of or relating to the heart.

cardiac arrest — a heart attack or when productive heart beating stops.

cardiovascular —pertaining to the heart and arteries.

cholesterol — a waxy fat present in some foods of animal origin; it is also manufacturered by the human body. Some cholesterol is needed by the body, but excessive amounts are associated with artery disease.

congestive heart failure — occurs when the heart is unable to pump well enough to maintain good circulation. It often occurs because of a weakness of the heart muscle due to disease or a mechanical fault in the valves that control the flow of blood.

coronary heart disease or coronary artery disease — narrowing or blockage of the coronary arteries which reduces the flow of blood to the heart muscle.

diastolic pressure — the pressure which remains in the blood vessels as the heart relaxes to allow for the flow of blood into its pumping chambers. The second number in a blood pressure reading.

diuretic — a drug that increases the flow of urine.

drug interaction — one drug or other substance increasing, decreasing or changing the effects of another drug.

edema — accumulation of fluid in the body.

EKG — see electrocardiograph.

electrocardiograph — a recording of the heart's electrical activity. By placing electrodes, usually with gel, on a person's arms, legs and chest the heart's electrical activity can be monitored and recorded onto a strip of graph paper.

fiber — dietary fiber, often called roughage, is the part of food that cannot be absorbed by the body. It is essential for proper elimination of body waste as it helps food move through the body. It is found in fruits, raw vegetables and whole grains. Highly processed foods, like white flour and sugar, contain little or no fiber.

generic name — the name given to the ingredient or ingredients in a drug as distinguished from brand names for drugs which may be trademarked by manufacturers.

heart attack — heart failure or abnormal, weak functioning of the heart after its blood supply is abruptly cut off, usually due to narrowing of the arteries or a blood clot.

high blood pressure — See hypertension.

hypertension — sustained high blood pressure of 140/90 or higher. The correct medical term for high blood pressure.

hypotension — low blood pressure.

kidney — located at the back of the abdomen, kidneys are responsible for filtering the blood and removing the waste materials. Normally people have two kidneys.

monounsaturated fats — fatty acids that have one double or triple bond per molecule. They are easily split and other substances can join them. Found in olive oil, chicken, almonds and some other nuts.

nephrology — the study of the kidneys.

obesity — being 20 to 40 percent heavier than your ideal weight.

oral contraceptive — a drug containing female hormones, usually synthetic estrogen and progesterone, to provide birth control by inhibiting the body's natural cycle of female hormone production which interferes with ovulation or the release of eggs.

polyunsaturated fats — fatty acids that have more than one double or triple bond per molecule. Found in fish, soybean, safflower, and corn oil. Polyunsaturated fats are usually soft or liquid at room temperature.

potassium — an essential mineral found in meat,

potatoes, raisins, nuts, tomatoes, banana, milk and fruit. It serves as an electrolyte in the body and plays a part in the regulation of blood pressure.

renin — a substance released into the blood by the kidney in response to stress that may change blood pressure.

salt — a common name for sodium chloride, a crystal solid chiefly used as a flavoring and a preservative. In the body, salt maintains fluid levels between the cells and the blood system and acts as an electrolyte to help chemical and electrical reactions.

saturated fat — a type of fat that raises blood cholesterol and trigylceride levels. All the atoms are joined by single bonds. Found in animal and dairy products such as beef, pork, lamb, veal, egg yolks, milk, butter, cheese, cream and a few vegetable fats, including coconut oil and hydrogenated vegetable shortening. Saturated fats are generally hard or solid at room temperature.

sphygmomanometer — an arm pressure cuff used to determine blood pressure.

stroke — an interruption of blood flow to an area of the brain, leading to damage and loss of function controlled by that area of the brain. Strokes can be caused by a blockage of a blood vessel in the brain or by bleeding from a blood vessel or an aneurysm into the brain. High blood pressure and smoking are the leading risk factors for stroke.

systolic pressure — the pressure which is produced as the heart contracts to pump blood out into the body. The first number in a blood pressure reading.

triglycerides — a type of fat carried throughout the body by the bloodstream: it is a particular combination of the three fatty acids. High trigylceride levels are associated with overeating, obesity, high-fat or high-sugar diets, diabetes and coronary artery disease. High levels are dangerous.

uremia — the build up of waste products in the blood, often associated with the progressive narrowing of the kidney blood vessels.

vein — any blood vessel that carries blood back to the heart from various parts of the body.

vitamin — organic chemical which is essential for normal chemical reactions in the body.

vitamin supplement — extra vitamins used to supplement or add to those found in the diet.

water pill —see diuretic.

Bibliography

Bennett, Cleaves M., M.D. *Control Your High Blood Pressure Without Drugs.* Garden City, NY.: Doubleday & Company, 1984.

Brams, William A. M.D. *How To Live With Your High Blood Pressure.* New York, NY.: Arco Publishing Co, 1973.

Chapman, Charles F. *Medical Dictionary for the Non-professional.* Woodbury, NY.: Barron's Educational Series, Inc., 1984.

Drugs of Choice from The Medical Letter. New Rochelle, NY.: The Medical Letter, Inc., 1985.

Cawood, Frank and Rita Warmack. *Arteries Cleaned Out Naturally.* Peachtree City, GA.: FC&A Publishing, 1986.

Failes, Janice McCall and Frank W. Cawood. *Encyclopedia of Little Known Secrets of Perfect Natural Health.* Peachtree City, GA.: FC&A Publishing, 1988.

Failes, Janice McCall and Frank W. Cawood. *Encyclopedia of Natural Health Secrets and Cures.* Peachtree City, GA.: FC&A Publishing, 1988.

Failes, Janice McCall and Frank W. Cawood. *Natural Healing Encyclopedia.* Peachtree City, GA.: FC&A Publishing, 1987.

Feinman, Max L. M.D. and Josleen Wilson. *Live Longer: Control Your Blood Pressure.* New York, NY.: Coward, McCann & Geoghegan, Inc., 1977.

Galton, Lawrence. *The Silent Disease: Hypertension.* New York, NY.: New American Library, 1974.

Shulman, Neil B. M.D., E. Saunders, M.D. and W. Hall, M.D. *High Blood Pressure.* New York, NY.: Macmillan Publishing Company, 1987.

Sorrentino, Sandy M.D., Ph.D., and Carl Hausman. *Coping With High Blood Pressure.* New York, NY.: Dembner Books, 1986.